AF440108

Theory and Practice of Chromatographic Techniques

Theory and Practice of Chromatographic Techniques

Sanjay B. Bari

M.Pharm. Ph.D. F.I.C.

Principal and Professor
H. R. Patel Institute of Pharmaceutical Education and Research,
Shirpur Dist-Dhule M.S. India.

Leonard L. Williams

M.S., Ph.D.

Director and Professor

Food Safety and Microbiology at the Center for Excellence in Post-Harvest
Technologies (CEPHT),. North Carolina Agricultural and Technical State
University. USA.

Yogini S. Jaiswal

M.Pharm., Ph.D.

Postdoctoral Research scholar

North Carolina Agricultural and Technical State University, USA.

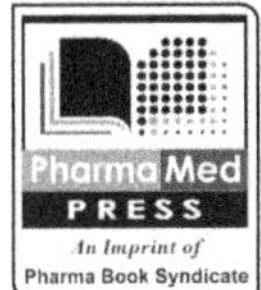

PharmaMed Press

An imprint of Pharma Book Syndicate

A unit of BSP Books Pvt. Ltd.
4-4-309/316, Giriraj Lane,
Sultan Bazar, Hyderabad - 500 095.

Theory and Practice of Chromatographic Techniques
by *Sanjay B. Bari, Leonard L. Williams, and Yogini S. Jaiswal*

Published by

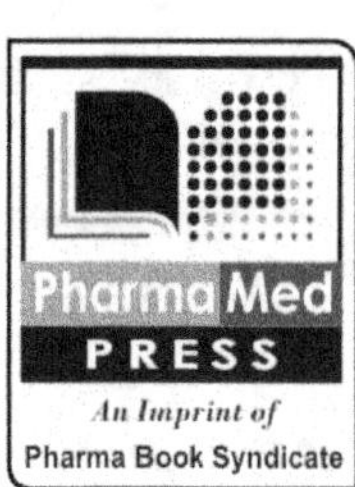

PharmaMed Press

An imprint of Pharma Book Syndicate
A unit of BSP Books Pvt. Ltd.
4-4-309/316, Giriraj Lane, Sultan Bazar, Hyderabad - 500 095.
Phone: 040-23445600, 23445688; Fax: 91+40-23445611
E-mail: info@pharmamedpress.com
www.pharmamedpress.com/pharmamedpress.net

ISBN: 978-93-5230-164-5 (Hardback)

CONTENTS

Chapter 1   **Analytical Methods – An Overview**

Chapter 2   **Basics of Chromatography**

Chapter 3   Preparative Chromatography

Chapter 4   Thin Layer Chromatography (TLC)

Chapter 5   High Performance Thin Layer Chromatography (HPTLC) and Hyphenated Techniques

PREFACE

Analytical chemistry and research in the field of Chromatography have witnessed an upsurge in their applications since the past few decades. Basics of chromatography have not only been an essential part of curriculum but also have formed the foundation for several budding researchers who gain an interest in this field from their University level education.

This book is designed with a view to provide insights into the fundamental principles and applications of different types of chromatography. There is a plentitude of books in this field; however few books are presented in this subject at undergraduate level. This book is particularly written considering undergraduate students as the target audience. Our aim is to facilitate understanding of chromatographic techniques to undergraduate students, through chapters designed in a lucid language.

The first chapter of this book provides an overview of analytical chemistry, followed by the second chapter which explains the history, nomenclature, and theories of chromatography. The following chapters detail Preparative Chromatography, Thin Layer Chromatography (TLC), High Performance Thin Layer Chromatography (HPTLC), High Performance Liquid Chromatography (HPLC), Gas Chromatography–Mass Spectrometry (GC-MS), Ionic Interaction Chromatography and Chiral Chromatography. The last chapter provides an overview of methods for Analysis of data obtained from Hyphenated Chromatography.

The field of chromatography is certainly immense and covering every aspect is beyond the scope of this book. However, this book is formulated to deliver comprehensive and substantial information for undergraduate students which will form their first step towards future research. We hope this book will accomplish its aim of serving as an aid to students for developing their understanding in the field of Chromatography. We welcome suggestions and constructive criticism from students and mentors in the subject that will help us improve the quality of this book in forthcoming editions.

- Authors

ACKNOWLEDGEMENTS

The book has been written by authors of this book, but it would have been an incomplete venture without the help of many sources and people related to this endeavor. We express our sincere thanks to the reviewers of this book that helped us to improve the quality of the text. We acknowledge the renowned authors of other books in this field who have served as an inspiration and source of guidance for this compilation. We extend our thanks to all our well-wishers and the publication team for drafting, copy editing and essential inputs in the final stages of the publication of our book. Finally, we thank our families for the encouragement and support during the writing of this book. Dr. Bari would like to thank the management of H. R. Patel Institute of Pharmaceutical Education and Research, Shirpur, Maharashtra for providing the facilities and co-operating during drafting of this book. The authors, Dr. Leonard Williams and Dr. Yogini Jaiswal acknowledge the support of North Carolina Agricultural and Technical State University, NC, USA, in providing its facilities and encouragement during drafting and editing of this book. We wish to contribute to serve the mission of the University, through exemplary instruction of students in science and technology related fields, worldwide.

- Authors

Analytical Methods – An Overview

Introduction

In many paradigms of analytical chemistry, it is necessary to have reliable and identical data on recovery, detection and quantification of drugs. In the pharmaceutical research laboratories, and industries the quality control and assessment **(QC & A)** parameters are required to examine and evaluate the quality, safety and efficacy of the products or formulations manufactured and analyzed. In clinical analysis, **(QC & A)** is a vital aspect of safety and patient care, diagnosis and control of therapy of individual patient, and for biological analysis.

Quality control and assessment **(QC & A)** forms an essential part of the instruments or automated systems used for production in laboratories and industries. For an *internal quality control* (IQC) a continued observation is required for everyday calibration of instruments. *External Quality Assessment* (EQA) serves an important part of assuring laboratory compliance. To comprehend, it is necessary to understand the basic concept of quality, quality assurance and quality control to apply these parameters of check to a range of instrumental methods and the methods developed therewith.

Quality is the entirety of features and uniqueness of a product or a service that bears on its capability to assure stated or implied needs.

Quality Assurance (QA) is a term used to illustrate the means of ensuring the precision of the results in a laboratory. It is an internal analytical tool that is concerned with the prevention of quality problems through planned and systematic activities.

Quality Control (QC) is a feature of **QA** that is concerned with the activities and techniques employed to achieve and maintain the product quality.

The aim of **QC** is to ensure conformity with the quality specifications and provide economic effectiveness at relevant stages of operation of an analytical method.

The requirements which are necessary for (**QC & A**) fall within the sphere of quality assurance program and to seek out for international quality standards, laboratories must function in accordance with (**ISO / IEC 17025: 2000**) (**ISO / IEC 2000**), *Good Laboratory Practices (***GLP; OECD 1992**) or the *Mandatory Health and Human Service Guidelines for federal workplace drug testing program* (**DHHS 1994**).

Aims of Analytical Chemistry

The basic requirement for the study of the chemical and biological properties of a given molecule is that the analyte sample should be homogeneous.

In 1894, Wilhelm Ostwald wrote "Analytical chemistry, or the art of recognizing different substances and determining their constituents, takes a prominent position among the applications of science, since the questions which it enables us to answer arise wherever chemical processes are employed for scientific or technical purposes."

The aims of analytical chemistry encompass the following:
1. The advancement of theory and development of scientific validation of the existing analytical methods.
2. Detailing the scientific basis of new analytical methods which help them comply with the requirements of advancing science and modern production.
3. Analysis of products from natural substances, environment and industrial materials.

Selection of Method of Analysis

The selection of an analytical method is dependent upon many factors, such as: chemical properties of an analyte and its concentration, sample matrix, speed and cost of analysis, type of analysis, i.e., quantitative or qualitative and the number of samples.

A *Qualitative Method* gives information about the identity of a particular analyte in a sample. A *Quantitative Method* yields information about the relative amounts of one or more analytes present in a sample. A separation process is generally an indispensable step for both a qualitative and a quantitative process.

Criteria for Selection of a Method

- The technical model/method/instrumentation that is compatible with the properties of the sample to be analysed must be present.

- The method must meet the particular standards of precision, sensitivity and specificity.

- Operating cost must remain within reasonable economic limits

- Before starting with the method development one must have knowledge about the nature of the sample; the objectives of analysis should be defined and the number of samples must be known. The nature of the sample helps one to decide or conclude about the best method to proceed with the method development. Generally, chemical analysis is performed only on a small division of the product/sample whose composition is to be studied. But, the composition of the small fraction taken for analysis must be identical to the composition of the bulk material. The procedure of acquiring a representative sample is called 'sampling'. Some products/ samples need pre-treatment prior to analysis in order to avoid interferences or to concentrate the analytes. The aims of a separation process for example should be precise and detailed before starting with a method development. It may for example, be necessary to resolve all the constituents of a sample or it may be required that the analytes are separated from impurities and degradation products without the need to further separate these impurities and degradation products from each other. The concluding process should meet all the requirements specified in the beginning of the method and when the method for quantitative use is finalized it should be validated.

Various Methods of Analysis

Since few decades, different methods of analysis are used for quantitative analyses which include:

Spectroscopic Methods:

- UV – Visible Spectroscopic Method
- Infrared Spectroscopy
- Mass Spectroscopy
- NMR Spectroscopic method

Spectrometry Method:

- Mass Spectrometry

Chromatographic Methods: Most widely used chromatographic methods include

- High Performance Liquid Chromatography **(HPLC)**
- High Performance Thin Layer Chromatography **(HPTLC)**
- Gas Chromatography (also sometimes called as Gas Liquid Chromatography-**GLC,** vapor-phase chromatography -**VPC,** or gas–liquid partition chromatography-**GLPC)**
- GC-MS
- LC-MS

Electrochemical Methods:

- Coulometry
- Voltametry
- Potentiometry
- Atomic Spectrometry
- Emission (plasma) Spectrometry
- Conductometry
- Polarography
- Amperometry

Other Methods:

- Gravimetry
- Titrimetry

Hyphenated Techniques Adding New Life into the Analytical Instrumentation

Widespread research in the fields of biochemistry, drug discovery, environmental testing, and even space research, has increased the need for high-performance analytical equipment. Each new development offers much more than its forerunner. Traditional analytical approaches including HPLC (High-Performance Liquid Chromatography), GC (Gas Chromatograph), UV (Ultraviolet) detection, etc., have become inadequate to efficiently address the challenges in analyses of species-specificity and sensitivity. Modern analyses methods, whose developments are referred to as hyphenated techniques, commence from the traditional use of specific detection.

Hyphenated Techniques combine chromatographic and spectral methods to exploit the advantages of both. Chromatography techniques produce pure or nearly pure fractions of chemical components in a mixture. Spectroscopic techniques produce selective information for identification using standards or library spectra.

Hyphenated techniques and instruments have been around for over 15-20 years now. The GC-MS (Mass Spectrophotometer), ICP-MS (Inductive Coupled Plasma – Mass Spectrophotometer) have been finding applications in several research efforts across various fields. Stand-alone instruments could analyze various physical properties such as boiling point, toxicity, solubility and metabolic pathways in different living organisms. With integrated such the HPLC-ICP-MS or the GC-ICP-MS, sample preparation before analysis is minimized and 'on-line' species separation is rapid. These integrated techniques are becoming increasingly popular in applications where analyses of complex matrices with low detection limits and high specificity are expected.

The hyphenated techniques offer advantages of, shorter analysis time, higher degree of automation, increased sample throughput, better reproducibility, reduction of contamination due to a closed system unit and enhanced combined selectivity and higher degree of information output.

Researchers in various fields are already using in varied applications and in the coming era research will be greatly benefited by these hyphenated techniques.

The proceeding chapters would help gain insights into Chromatography, its basic principles and related hyphenated techniques which are of paramount importance in the field of analytical research worldwide.

2 Basics of Chromatography

History

Almost all substances, one comes in contact with on a daily basis are impure or more appropriately said are mixtures of more than one component. Similarly, compounds synthesized or extracted in the research laboratories are rarely produced pure. As a result, a major focus of research is designing methods of separating and identifying components of mixtures.

Many separation techniques are based upon the physical differences between the components of a mixture. For example, filtration relies upon the fact of substances being present in different states (solid vs. liquid); centrifugation depends upon the differences in density; and distillation is carried out based on the differences in boiling points of the various components. Chromatography makes use of differences in solubility and adsorption for separation of substances.

The word chromatography is derived from two Greek words "*Chroma*" and "*graphein*" literally meaning "color" and "writing". The history of chromatography dates back to the mid-19th century to the 21st century. Chromatography, literally "color writing", was used and named in the first decade of the 20th century, primarily for the separation of plant leaves pigments such as chlorophyll (which is green), carotenoids and xanthophylls (which are orange and yellow).

The earliest use of chromatography was done by passing a solution containing mixture of various substances through an inert material to create separation of the components in the solution based on differential adsorption. This work is sometimes credited to German chemist Friedlieb Ferdinand Runge. He was the one who in 1855 described the use of paper to analyze dyes. Runge dropped different inorganic chemicals in the form of circular spots on a filter paper already impregnated with another chemical, and reactions between the different chemicals created unique color patterns. However according to historical analysis of L. S. Ettre, Runge's work was said to be irrelevant to chromatography and was instead considered to be a precursor of chemical spot tests such as the Schiff test.

In the 1860s, Christian Friedrich Schönbein and his student Friedrich Goppelsroeder published the first experiments they carried as an attempt to study the different rates at which different substances move through filter paper. Schönbein, formed the basis for the technique capillary analysis, who thought that capillary action (rather than adsorption) was responsible for the movement of components on filter paper. Goppelsroeder used capillary analysis to test the movement rates of a wide variety of substances. Distinct from the modern paper chromatography, capillary analysis technique used reservoirs of the substance being analyzed, and overlapping zones of the solution components rather than separate points or bands were observed.

Work on capillary analysis continued, but without much technical advancement, until the 20th century. The first important advancement over Goppelsroeder's methods came with the work of Raphael E. Liesegang. In 1927, Raphael placed filter strips in closed containers saturated by solvent's vapors. In 1943 he used discrete spots of sample adsorbed to filter paper, and dipped them in pure solvent to achieve separation. This method, fundamentally similar to modern paper chromatography, was published just before the independent and far more significant work of Archer Martin and his collaborators that established the extensive use of paper chromatography for analysis.

Mikhail Tsvet's Contribution to Chromatography

The first true chromatography is credited to the Russian botanist Mikhail Tsvet. Tsvet applied his observations of filter paper extraction to the method of column fractionation that had been developed in the 1890s for separating the constituents of petroleum. He separated yellow, orange, and green plant pigments (which are known today as xanthophylls, carotenes, and chlorophylls, respectively) by using a liquid-adsorption column containing calcium carbonate. The method was first printed and described in 1903, in the proceedings of the Warsaw Society of Naturalists, section of biology. He used the term *chromatography* for the first time in print in 1906 in his two papers about chlorophyll in the German botanical journal, *Berichte der Deutschen Botanischen Gesellschaft*. In 1907 Mikhail Tsvet demonstrated his chromatograph for the German Botanical Society.

In one of his lectures published in 1905, Tsvet described using filter paper to estimate the properties of plant pigments in his experiments. He found that different pigments of plants required solvents of different polarity in order to be extracted. He extracted some pigments (like orange carotenes and yellow xanthophylls) with non-polar solvents, and other pigments (such as chlorophyll) required polar solvents. He justified the reason behind this result that chlorophyll was strongly bonded to the plant tissue by adsorption, and hence stronger solvents were necessary to overcome the adsorption. To examine this, he applied liquified pigments to filter paper, allowed the spots to dry, and then applied various solvents to observe which could extract the pigments. He observed the same pattern as from leaf extractions carried out earlier. Carotene could be extracted using non-polar solvents, but chlorophyll required polar solvents for extraction. However, Tsvet's work received less application and consideration until the 1930s.

Martin and Synge's Contribution to Partition Chromatography

Chromatography methods remained much unchanged after Tsvet's work until the outburst of mid-20th century research in advanced techniques. The success is particularly credited to the work of Archer John Porter Martin and Richard Laurence Millington Synge. By the association of chromatography and that of countercurrent solvent extraction, Martin and Synge developed partition chromatography to separate chemicals with only slight differences in partition between two liquid solvents. Martin, who had been working previously in vitamin chemistry, collaborated with Synge in 1938. Together, they designed an equipment to separate amino acids. Their experiments with countercurrent extraction machines and liquid-liquid chromatography methods were unsuccessful in spite of several attempts. Martin then came up with the idea of packing columns with silica gel to hold water stationary while an organic solvent is passed through the column. Martin and Synge demonstrated the method by separating amino acids bands in the column by the addition of methyl red. Later, in a number of publications starting from 1941, they published very important methods of separating amino acids and other organic chemicals.

In search of improved and easier methods of identifying the amino acid constituents of peptides, Martin and Synge switched to other chromatography media's. They published a short abstract in 1943 followed by a detailed article in 1944 which describes the use of filter paper as the stationary phase for separating amino acids i.e, now termed as paper chromatography. Martin, Synge and their collaborators applied paper chromatography in the year 1947, (along with Fred Sanger's reagent for identifying N-terminal residues) to determine the pentapeptide sequence of *Gramicidin S.* These experiments and related paper chromatography methods formed the foundations to Fred Sanger's attempt of determining the amino acid sequence of insulin.

Based on the principles which Martin and Synge had published in 1941 paper, Martin worked in collaboration with Anthony T. James and developed gas chromatography method in the beginning of 1949. In 1952, Martin received a Nobel Prize in Chemistry (shared with Synge, for their previous chromatography work). In the lecture while receiving the Nobel prize, Martin announced the successful separation of a wide variety of natural compounds by gas chromatography.

The ease and efficiency of gas chromatography technique for separating organic chemicals drove the rapid adoption of the method. It gave a boost to the fast development of new detection methods for analyzing the output. The thermal conductivity detector, described in 1954 by N. H. Ray, formed the basis for development of several other methods. The contributions of Martin and Synge set the phase for high performance liquid chromatography.

The initial steps in thin layer chromatography took place in the 1940s, and techniques advanced speedily in the 1950s after the beginning of comparatively larger plates and fairly stable materials for sorbent layers.

Nomenclature for Chromatography

The original activities of the International Union of Pure and Applied Chemistry (IUPAC) Commission on Analytical Nomenclature aimed to create a unified nomenclature applicable to all forms of chromatography, took place over 20 years ago. Since that time chromatographic techniques have advanced significantly. The present nomenclature was prepared by Dr. L. S. Ettre originally for the Commission on Analytical Nomenclature. The present nomenclature deals with all chromatographic terms and definitions used in the major chromatographic techniques such as gas, liquid and supercritical-fluid chromatography, column and planar chromatography, partition, adsorption, ion-exchange and exclusion chromatography. However, it does not include terms related to the results calculated from chromatography data such as e.g., the various molecular weight terms computed from the primary data obtained by exclusion chromatography, Also it does not deal with detailed information related to detection and detectors or the relationships between chemical structure and chromatographic retention.

Method for separating the components, or solutes, of a mixture on the basis of the relative amounts of each solute distributed between a moving fluid, called the mobile phase, and an adjacent stationary phase. The mobile phase may be either a liquid or a gas, while the stationary phase is either a solid or a liquid.

Basic Definitions

- *Chromatography*

  Chromatography is a physical method of separation in which the components to be separated are distributed between two phases, one of which is stationary (stationary phase) while the other (the mobile phase) moves in a definite direction.

- *Chromatogram*

  A graphical or other presentation of detector response, concentration of analyte in the effluent or other quantity used as a measure of effluent concentration versus effluent volume or time. In planar chromatography "chromatogram" may refer to the paper or layer with the separated zones.

- *Chromatograph*

  The assembly of apparatus for carrying out chromatographic separation.

- *Stationary Phase*

  The stationary phase is one of the two phases forming a chromatographic system. It may be a solid, a gel or a liquid. If a liquid, it may be distributed on a solid. This solid may or may not contribute to the separation process. The liquid may also be chemically bonded to the solid *(Bonded Phase)* or immobilized onto it *(Immobilized Phase)*.

The expression ***Chromatographic Bed*** or ***Sorbent*** may be used as a general term to denote any of the different forms in which the stationary phase is used.

Particularly in gas chromatography where the stationary phase is most often a liquid, the term ***Liquid Phase*** is used for it as compared to the ***Gas Phase,*** i.e., the mobile phase. However, particularly in the early development of liquid chromatography, the term "liquid phase" had also been used to characterize the mobile phase as compared to the "solid phase" i.e., the stationary phase. Due to this ambiguity, the use of the term "liquid phase" is discouraged. If the physical state of the stationary phase is to be expressed, the use of the adjective forms such as ***Liquid Stationary Phase*** and ***Solid Stationary Phase,*** ***Bonded Phase*** or ***Immobilized Phase*** is proposed.

- ***Bonded Phase***

  A stationary phase which is covalently bonded to the support particles or to the inside wall of the column tubing.

- ***Immobilized Phase***

  A stationary phase which is immobilized on the support particles, or on the inner wall of the column tubing, e.g., by in situ polymerization (cross-linking) after coating.

- ***Mobile Phase***

  A fluid which percolates through or along the stationary bed, in a definite direction. It may be a liquid ***(Liquid Chromatography)*** or a gas ***(Gas Chromatography)*** or a supercritical fluid ***(Supercritical-Fluid Chromatography).*** In gas chromatography, the expression ***Carrier Gas*** may be used for the mobile phase. In elution chromatography the expression ***Eluent*** is also used for the mobile phase.

- ***Elute*** (verb)

  To chromatograph by elution chromatography. The process of elution may be stopped while all the sample components are still on the chromatographic bed or continued until the components have left the chromatographic bed.

The term "elute" is referred to the term Develop used in former nomenclatures of planar chromatography.

- *Efluent*

  The mobile phase leaving the column is called efluent.

- *Sample*

  The mixture consisting of a number of components, the separation of which is attempted on the chromatographic bed as they are carried or eluted by the mobile phase is the sample.

- *Sample Components*

  They are chemically pure constituents of the sample. They may be un-retained (i.e., not delayed) by the stationary phase, partially retained (i.e., eluted at different times) or retained permanently.

  The terms Elute or Analyte are also acceptable for a sample component.

- *Solute*

  A term referring to the sample components in partition chromatography.

- *Solvent*

  A term sometimes referring to the liquid stationary phase in partition chromatography.

  Note: In liquid chromatography the term "solvent" has been often used for the mobile phase.

  This usage is not recommended.

- *Zone*

  A region in the chromatographic bed where one or more components of the sample are located. The term Band may also be used for it.

Principal Methods

- *Frontal Chromatography*

  A procedure in which the sample (liquid or gas) is fed continuously into the chromatographic bed. In frontal chromatography no additional mobile phase is used.

- *Displacement Chromatography*

  A procedure in which the mobile phase contains a compound (the Displacer) more strongly retained than the components of the sample under examination. The sample is fed into the system as a finite slug.

- ***Elution Chromatography***

  A procedure in which the mobile phase is continuously passed through or along the chromatographic bed and the sample is fed into the system as a finite slug.

Classification according to the Shape of the Chromatographic Bed

- ***Column Chromatography***

  A separation technique in which the stationary bed is within a tube. The particles of the solid stationary phase or the support coated with a liquid stationary phase may fill the whole inside volume of the tube (Packed Column) or be concentrated on or along the inside tube wall leaving an open, unrestricted path for the mobile phase in the middle part of the tube (Open-Tubular Column).

- ***Planar Chromatography***

  A separation technique in which the stationary phase is present as or on a plane. The plane can be a paper, serving as such or impregnated by a substance as the stationary bed (Paper Chromatography, PC) or a layer of solid particles spread on a support, e.g., a glass plate (Thin Layer Chromatography, TLC). Sometimes planar chromatography is also termed Open-Bed Chromatography.

Classification according to the Physical State of the Mobile Phase

Chromatographic techniques are often classified by specifying the physical state of ***both*** phases used. Accordingly, the following terms are in use:

Gas-liquid chromatography (GLC)

Gas-solid chromatography (GSC)

Liquid-liquid chromatography (LLC)

Liquid-solid chromatography (LSC)

The term ***Gas-Liquid Partition Chromatography*** (GLPC) can also be found in the literature.

However, often distinction between these modes is not easy. For example, in GC, a liquid maybe used to modify an adsorbent-type solid stationary phase.

- ***Gas Chromatography (GC)***

  A separation technique in which the mobile phase is a gas. Gas chromatography is always carried out in a column.

- ***Liquid Chromatography (LC)***

  A separation technique in which the mobile phase is a liquid. Liquid chromatography can be carried out either in a column or on a plane. Present-day liquid chromatography generally utilizing very small particles and a relatively high inlet pressure is often Characterized by the term High-Performance or (High-pressure) Liquid Chromatography, and the acronym HPLC.

- ***Supercritical-Fluid Chromatography (SFC)***

  A separation technique in which the mobile phase is a fluid above and relatively close to its critical temperature and pressure. In general the terms and definitions used in gas or liquid chromatography are equally applicable to supercritical-fluid chromatography.

Classification according to the Mechanism of Separation

- ***Adsorption Chromatography***

  Separation is based mainly on differences between the adsorption affinities of the sample components for the surface of an active solid. The separation in this type of chromatography is based upon the differences in polarity between the solute components and the stationary phase. The polar molecules get strongly adsorbed by a polar stationary phase and the non-polar molecules; get strongly adsorbed by non-polar stationary phase.

  In a surface adsorption chromatography process, the solute components compete for adsorption sites on a stationary phase. A diagram indicating various mechanisms of chromatographic separation is shown in Fig. 2.1.

  The choice of adsorbent is based upon the polarity of the solute components to be separated.

The selection of mobile phase is equally crucial task. The polarity of the mobile phase should be selected such that it complements the choice of stationary phase.

- ***Partition Chromatography***

  Separation is based mainly on differences between the solubilities of the sample components in the stationary phase (gas chromatography), or on differences between the solubilities of the components in the mobile and stationary phases (liquid chromatography).

  In partition chromatography, a solid support such as silica gel, cellulose powder, or kieselguhr (hydrated silica) is coated with a stationary liquid phase. The solute components move depending upon their relative solubilities in the stationary and mobile phases.

  A low degree of mutual solubility is desirable between the coated liquid stationary phase and the mobile phase. Hydrophilic stationary phase liquids are used in combination with hydrophobic mobile phases which is termed as "normal-phase chromatography".

- ***Ion-Exchange Chromatography***

  Separation is based mainly on differences in the ion exchange affinities of the sample components. Present day ion-exchange chromatography on small particle high efficiency columns and usually utilizing conductometric or spectroscopic detectors is often referred to as Ion Chromatography (IC).

  In this type of chromatography, the stationary phase consists of an insoluble porous resinous material that contains fixed charge-carrying groups. Counter-ions are loosely complexed with such groups. There is a reversible exchange of these ions when the mobile phase containing ionised or partially ionised molecules of the same charge as the counter-ions moves through the stationary phase bed. The degree of separation between the solute components depends upon the degree of affinity between the stationary phase and solute.

- ***Exclusion Chromatography***

  Separation is based mainly on exclusion effects, such as differences in molecular size and/or shape or charge. The term Size-Exclusion Chromatography may also be used when separation is based on molecular size. The terms Gel Filtration and Gel-Permeation Chromatography (GPC) were used earlier to describe this process when the stationary phase is a swollen gel. The term Ion-Exclusion

Chromatography is specifically used for the separation of ions in an aqueous phase.

- *Affinity Chromatography*

  This expression characterizes the particular variant of chromatography in which the unique biological specificity of the analyte and ligand interaction is utilized for the separation.

Special Techniques

- *Reversed-Phase Chromatography*

  An elution procedure used in liquid chromatography in which the mobile phase is significantly more polar then the stationary phase, e.g., a microporous silica-based material with chemicallybonded alkyl chains. The term "reverse phase" is an incorrect expression which is to be avoided.

- *Normal-Phase Chromatography*

  An elution procedure in which the stationary phase is more polar than the mobile phase. This term is used in liquid chromatography to emphasize the contrast to reversed-phase chromatography.

- *Isocratic Analysis*

  The procedure in which the composition of the mobile phase remains constant during the elution process.

- *Gradient Elution*

  The procedure in which the composition of the mobile phase is changed continuously or stepwise during the elution process.

- *Stepwise Elution*

  The elution process in which the composition of the mobile phase is changed in steps during a single chromatographic run.

- *Two-Dimensional Chromatography*

  A procedure in which parts or all of the separated sample components are subjected to additional separation steps. This can be done e.g., by conducting a particular fraction eluting from the column into another column (system) having different separation characteristics. When combined with additional separation steps, this may be described as Multi-Dimensional Chromatography.

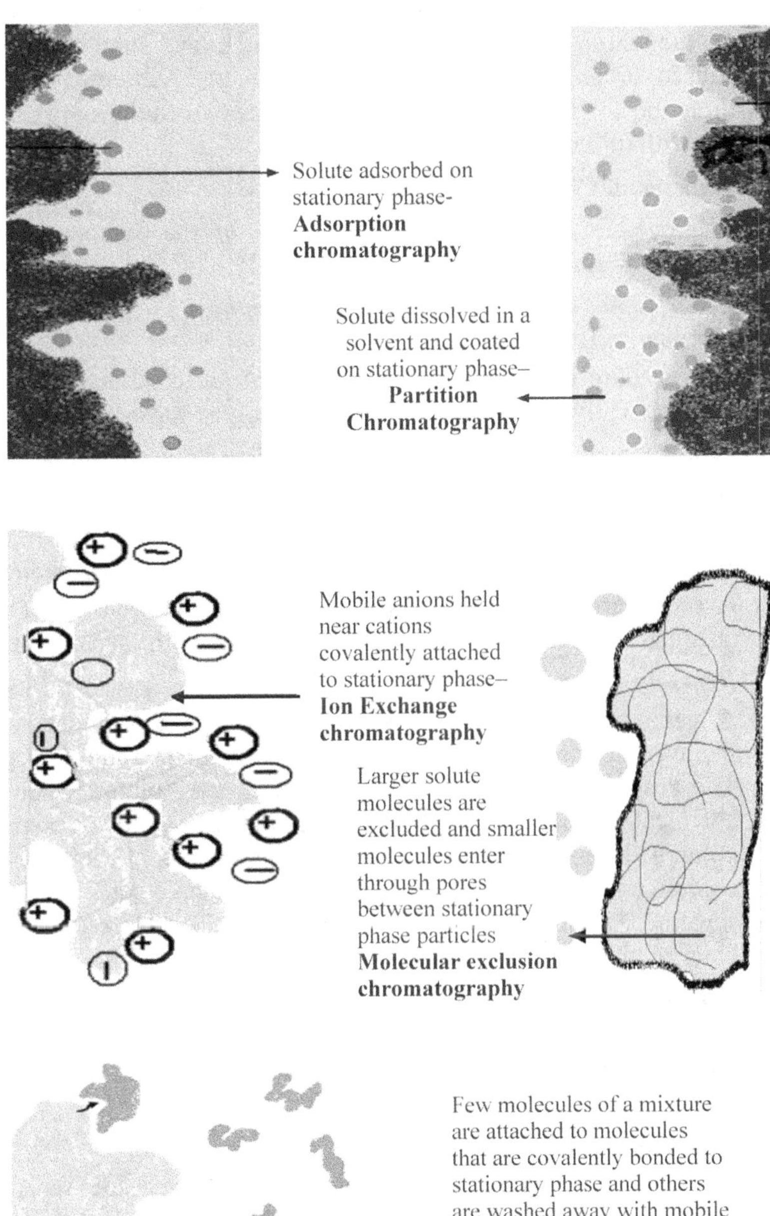

Figure 2.1 Classification of chromatographic methods according to the mechanism of separation

In planar chromatography two-dimensional chromatography refers to the chromatographic process in which the components are caused to migrate first in one direction and subsequently in a direction at right angles to the first one; the two elutions are carried out with different eluents.

- ***Isothermal Chromatography***

A procedure in which the temperature of the column is kept constant during the separation.

- ***Programmed-Temperature Chromatography (Temperature Programming)***

A procedure in which the temperature of the column is changed systematically during a part or the whole of the separation.

- ***Programmed-Flow Chromatography (Flow Programming)***

A procedure in which the rate of flow of the mobile phase is changed systematically during a part or the whole of the separation.

- ***Programmed-Pressure Chromatography (Pressure Programming)***

A procedure in which the inlet pressure of the mobile phase is changed systematically during a part or whole of the separation.

- ***Reaction Chromatography***

A technique in which the identities of the sample components are intentionally changed between sample introduction and detection. The reaction can take place upstream of the column when the chemical identity of the individual components passing through the column differs from that of the original sample, or between the column and the detector when the original sample components are separated in the column but their identity is changed prior to entering the detection device.

- ***Pyrolysis-Gas Chromatography***

A version of reaction chromatography in which a sample is thermally decomposed to simpler fragments before entering the column.

- ***Post-Column Derivatisation***

A version of reaction chromatography in which the separated sample components eluting from the column are derivatized prior to entering the detector. The derivatisation process is generally carried out "on-the-fly", i.e., during transfer of the sample components from the column to the detector. Derivatisation may also be carried out before the sample enters the column or the planar medium; this is pre-column (preliminary) Derivatisation.

Terms Related to the Chromatographic System
Apparatus in Column Chromatography

- ***Pump***

  A device designed to deliver the mobile phase at a controlled flow-rate to the separation system. Pumps are generally used in liquid chromatography.

- ***Syringe Pumps***

  Pumps with a piston, which advances at a controlled rate within a smooth cylinder to displace the mobile phase.

- ***Reciprocating Pumps***

  Pumps with a single or multiple chamber, from which the mobile phase is displaced by reciprocating piston(s) or diaphragm(s).

- ***Pneumatic Pumps***

  Pumps which employ a gas to displace the liquid mobile phase either directly or via a piston.

- ***Sample Injector***

  A device by which a liquid, solid or gaseous sample is introduced into the mobile phase or the chromatographic bed.

- ***Direct Injector***

  A device which directly introduces the sample into the mobile-phase stream.

- ***Bypass Injector***

  A device in which the sample is first introduced into a chamber (loop), temporarily isolated from the mobile phase system by valves, which can be switched to make an instantaneous diversion of the mobile phase stream through the chamber to carry the sample to the column. A bypass injector may also be known as a Valve Injector or Sampling Valve.

- ***On-Column Injector***

  A device in which the sample is directly introduced into the column. In gas chromatography the on-column injector permits the introduction of the liquid sample into the column without prior evaporation.

- ***Flash Vaporizer***

  A heated device used in gas chromatography. Here the liquid sample is introduced into the carrier gas stream with simultaneous evaporation and mixing with the carrier gas prior to entering the column.

- ***Split Injection***

  A sample introduction technique used in gas chromatography. The sample is flash vaporized and after thorough mixing of the sample with the carrier gas, the stream is split into two portions, one being conducted to the column and the other being discarded.

- ***Programmed Temperature Vaporizer (PTV)***

  A sample introduction device used in gas chromatography. The liquid sample is introduced, usually with a syringe, into a device similar to a flash vaporizer, the temperature of which is kept low, below the boiling point of the sample components. After withdrawal of the syringe, the device is heated up very rapidly in a controlled fashion to evaporate the sample into the continuously flowing carrier gas stream. The PTV may also be used in the split mode: in this case, the carrier gas stream containing the evaporated sample components is split into two portions, one of which is conducted into the column while the other is discarded.

- ***Gas Sampling Valve***

  A bypass injector permitting the introduction of a gaseous sample of a given volume into a gas chromatograph.

- ***Column Oven***

  A thermostatically controlled oven containing the column, the temperature of which (Separation Temperature or Column Temperature) can be varied within a wide range.

- ***Fraction Collector***

  A device for recovering fractional volumes of the column effluent.

- ***Detector***

  A device that measures the change in the composition of the eluent by measuring physical or chemical properties.

Apparatus in Planar Chromatography

- ***Spotting Device***

  The syringe or micropipette used to deliver a fixed volume of sample as a spot or streak to the paper or thin-layer media at the origin.

- *Elution Chamber (Developing Chamber)*

  A closed container, the purpose of which is to enclose the media used as well as the mobile phase to maintain a constant environment in the vapor phase.

- *Sandwich Chamber*

  A chamber in which the walls are close enough to the paper or plate to provide a relatively fast equilibration.

- *Ascending Elution (Ascending Development)*

  A mode of operation in which the paper or plate is in a vertical or slanted position and the mobile phase is supplied to its lower edge; the upward movement depends on capillary action.

- *Horizontal Elution (Horizontal Development)*

  A mode of operation in which the paper or plate is in a horizontal position and the mobile-phase movement along the plane depends on capillary action.

- *Descending Elution (Descending Development)*

  A mode of operation in which the mobile phase is supplied to the upper edge of the paper or plate and the downward movement is governed mainly by gravity.

- *Radial Elution (Radial Development) or Circular Elution (Circular Development)*

  A mode of operation in which the sample is spotted at a point source at or near the middle of the plane and is carried outward in a circle by the mobile phase, also applied at that place.

- *Anticircular Elution (Anticircular Development)*

  Here the sample as well as the mobile phase is applied at the periphery of a circle and both move towards the center.

- *Chamber Saturation (Saturated Development)*

  This expression refers to the uniform distribution of the mobile phase vapour through the elution chamber prior to chromatography.

- *Unsaturated Elution (Unsaturated Development)*

  This expression refers to chromatography in an elution chamber without attaining chamber saturation.

- *Equilibration*

  The expression refers to the level of saturation of the chromatographic bed by the mobile-phase vapor prior to chromatography.

- *Visualization Chamber*

  A device in which the planar media may be viewed under controlled-wavelength light, perhaps after spraying with chemical reagents to render the separated components as visible spots under specified conditions.

- *Densitometer*

  A device which allows portions of the developed paper or thin-layer media to be scanned with a beam of light of a specified wavelength for measurements of UV or visible light absorption or fluorescence, providing values which can be used for the quantitation of the separated compounds.

Terms Related to the Chromatographic Process and the Theory of Chromatography

The Chromatographic Medium

- *Active Solid*

  A solid with sorptive properties.

- *Modified Active Solid*

  An active solid the sorptive properties of which have been changed by some treatment.

- *Solid Support*

  A solid that holds the stationary phase but, ideally, does not contribute to the separation process.

- *Binders*

  Additives used to hold the solid stationary phase to the inactive plate or sheet in thin-layer chromatography.

- *Gradient Layer*

  The chromatographic bed used in thin-layer chromatography in which there is a gradual transition in some property.

- *Impregnation*

  The modification of the separation properties of the chromatographic bed used in planar chromatography by appropriate additives.

- *Packing*

  The active solid, stationary liquid plus solid support, or swollen gel contained in a tube.

- ***Totally Porous Packing***

  Here the stationary phase permeates each porous particle.

- ***Pellicular Packing***

  In this case the stationary phase forms a porous outer shell on an impermeable particle.

- ***Particle Diameter (d_p)***

  The average diameter of the solid particles.

- ***Pore Radius (r_p)***

  The average radius of the pores within the solid particles.

- ***Liquid-Phase Loading***

  A term used in partition chromatography to express the relative amount of the liquid stationary phase in the column packing. It is equal to the mass fraction (%) of liquid stationary phase in the total packing (liquid stationary phase plus support).

The Column

- ***Column***

  The tube and the stationary phase contained within, through which the mobile phase passes.

- ***Packed Column***

  A tube containing a solid packing.

- ***Open-Tubular Column***

  A column, usually having a small diameter in which either the inner tube wall, or a liquid or active solid held stationary on the tube wall acts as the stationary phase and there is an open, unrestricted path for the mobile phase.

- ***Wall-Coated Open-Tubular (WCOT) Column***

  In these columns the liquid stationary phase is coated on the essentially unmodified smooth inner wall of the tube.

- ***Porous-Layer Open-Tubular (PLOT) Column***

  In these columns there is a porous layer on the inner wall. Porosity can be achieved by either chemical means (e.g., etching) or by the deposition of porous particles on the wall from asuspension. The porous layer may serve as a support for a liquid stationary phase or as the stationary phase itself.

- ***Support-Coated Open-Tubular (SCOT) Column***

  A version of a PLOT column in which the porous layer consists of support particles and was deposited from a suspension.

- ***Capillary Column***

  A general term for columns having a small diameter. A capillary column may contain a packingor have the stationary phase supported on its inside wall. The former case corresponds to Packed Capillary Column while the latter case corresponds to an Open-Tubular Column. Due to theambiguity of this term its use without an adjective is discouraged.

- ***Column Volume (V_c)***

  The geometric volume of the part of the tube that contains the packing:

  $$V_c = A_c L$$

  Where A_c is the internal cross-sectional area of the tube and L is the length of the packed part ofthe column.

  In the case of wall-coated open-tubular columns the column volume corresponds to the geometric volume of the whole tube having a liquid or a solid stationary phase on its wall.

- ***Bed Volume***

  Synonymous with Column Volume for a packed column.

- ***Column Diameter (d_c)***

  The inner diameter of the tubing.

- ***Column Radius (r_c)***

  The inside radius of the tubing.

- ***Column Length (l_c)***

  The length of that part of the tube which contains the stationary phase.

- ***Cross-Sectional Area of the Column (A_c)***

  The cross-sectional area of the empty tube:

  $$A_c = \pi r_c^2 = (\pi d_c / 2)^2$$

- ***Interparticle Volume of the Column (V_o)***

  The volume occupied by the mobile phase between the particles in the packed section of a column. It is also called the Interstitial Volume or the Void Volume of the column. In liquid chromatography, the interparticle volume is equal to the mobile-phase holdup volume (V_M) in the ideal case, neglecting any extra-column volume. In gas chromatography, the symbol V_G may be used for the interparticle volume of the column.

In the ideal case, neglecting any extra-column volume, V_G is equal to the corrected gas hold-upvolume (V_M^O) :

$$V_G = V_M^O = V_M . j$$

Where j, is Mobile Phase Compressibility Correction Factor (j). It is a factor, applying to a homogeneously filled column of uniform diameter, that corrects for the compressibility of the mobile phase in the column. It is also called the Compressibility Correction Factor.

- **Interparticle Porosity (ε)**

The interparticle volume of a packed column per unit column volume:

$$\varepsilon = V_0 / V_C$$

It is also called the Interstitial Fraction of the column.

- **Extra-column Volume**

The volume between the effective injection point and the effective detection point, excluding the part of the column containing the stationary phase. It is composed of the volumes of the injector, connecting lines and detector.

- **Dead-Volume**

This term is also used to express the extra-column volume. Strictly speaking, the term "dead-volume" refers to volumes within the chromatographic system which are not swept by the mobile phase. On the other hand, mobile phase is flowing through most of the extra-column volumes. Due to this ambiguity the use of the term "dead-volume" is discouraged.

- **Liquid-Phase Film Thickness (d_f)**

A term used in connection with open-tubular columns to express the average thickness of the liquid stationary phase film coated on the inside wall of the tubing.

- **Stationary-Phase Volume (V_s)**

The volume of the liquid stationary phase or the active solid in the column. The volume of any solid support is not included. In the case of partition chromatography with a liquid stationary phase, it is identical to the Liquid-Phase Volume (V_L).

- *Mass (Weight) of the Stationary Phase (W_s)*

The mass (weight) of the liquid stationary phase or the active solid in the column. The mass (weight) of any solid support is not included. In the case of partition chromatography with a liquid stationary phase it is identical to the Liquid Phase Mass (weight) (W_L).

- *Phase Ratio (β)*

The ratio of the volume of the mobile phase to that of the stationary phase in a column:

$$\beta = V_0 / V_C$$

In the case of open-tubular columns the geometric internal volume of the tube (V_C) is to be substituted for V_o

- *Specific Permeability (B_o)*

A term expressing the resistance of an empty tube or packed column to the flow of a fluid (the mobile phase). In the case of a packed column

$$B_o = d\,p^2\,\varepsilon^{\,3} / 180\,(1-\varepsilon)^2 \approx d\,p^2 / 1000$$

In the case of an open-tubular column

$$B_o = r_c^{\,2} / 8$$

- *Flow Resistance Parameter (Φ)*

This term is used to compare packing density and permeability of columns packed with different particles; it is dimensionless.

$$\Phi = d\,p^2 / B_o$$

where *dp* is the average particle diameter. In open-tubular columns $\Phi = 32$.

The Chromatogram

- *Differential Chromatogram*

A chromatogram obtained with a differential detector (see Fig. 2.2A).

- *Integral Chromatogram*

A chromatogram obtained with an integral detector (see Fig. 2.2B).

- ***Starting Point or Line***

  The point or line on a chromatographic paper or layer where the substance to be chromatographed is applied (P in Fig. 2.3).

- ***Spot***

  A zone in paper and thin-layer chromatography of approximately circular appearance.

- ***Spot Diameter (ST in Fig 2.3)***

  The width of the sample component spot before or after chromatography.

- ***Baseline***

  The portion of the chromatogram recording the detector response when only the mobile phase emerges from the column.

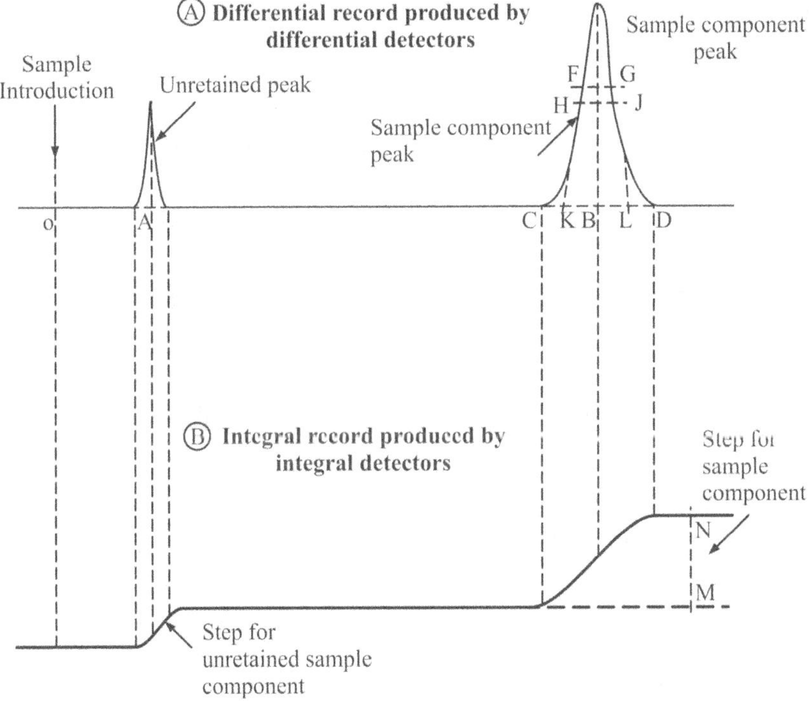

Figure 2.2 Typical chromatogram: **A.** Differential record produced by differential detector; **B.** Integralrecord produced by integral detector

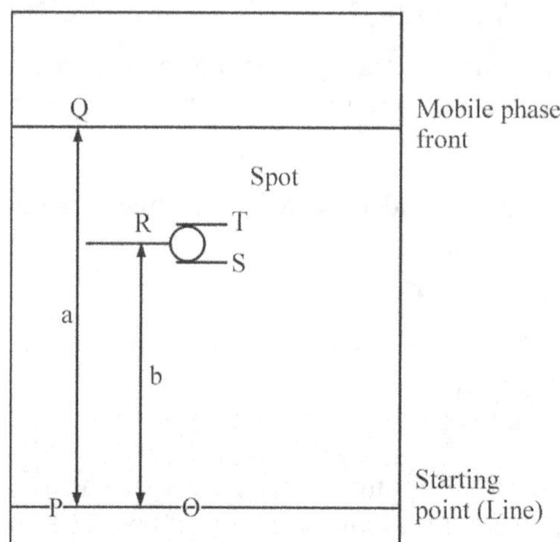

Figure 2.3 Typical planar chromatogram

- *Peak*

  The portion of a differential chromatogram recording the detector response when a single component is eluted from the column (see Fig. 2.2A). If separation is incomplete, two or more components may be eluted as one Unresolved Peak.

- *Peak Base (CD in Fig. 2.2A)*

  The interpolation of the baseline between the extremities of the peak.

- *Peak Area (CHFEGJD in Fig. 2.2A)*

  The area enclosed between the peak and the peak base.

- *Peak Maximum (E in Fig. 2.2A)*

  The point on the peak at which the distance to the peak base, measured in a direction parallel to the axis representing detector response, is a maximum.

- *Peak Height (EB in Fig. 2.2A)*

  The distance between the peak maximum and the peak base, measured in a direction parallel to the axis representing detector response.

- *Standard Deviation (σ)*

  The term in the exponent of the equation relating the width and height of a Gaussian peak:

$$y = y_o \cdot \exp. - \left[\frac{x^2}{2\sigma^2} \right]$$

where y is the peak height at any point on the peak, y_o is the peak height at maximum, x is the distance from the ordinate (i.e., half of the width at that point), and σ is the standard deviation of the peak. In practice, the standard deviation can be calculated from one of the peak-width values specified below.

- ***Variance of the Peak***

  The square of the standard deviation (σ^2)

- ***Peak-Widths***

  Peak-widths represent retention dimensions (time or volume) parallel to the baseline. If the baseline is not parallel to the axis representing time or volume, then the peak-widths are to be drawn parallel to this axis. Three peak-width values are commonly used in chromatography (see Fig. 2.2A and Fig. 2.4).

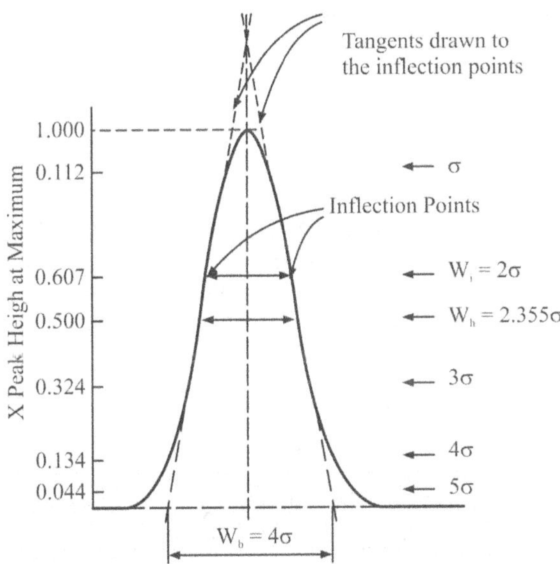

Figure 2.4 Widths of a Gaussian peak at various heights, as a function of the standard deviation of the peak

- ***Peak-Width at Base (W_b) (KL in Fig.2.2A and Fig. 2.4)***

  The segment of the peak base intercepted by the tangents drawn to the inflection points on eitherside of the peak.

- ***Peak-Width at Half Height (W$_h$) (HJ in Fig.2.2A and Fig.2.4)***

  The length of the line parallel to the peak base at 50% of the peak height that terminates at the intersection with the two limbs of the peak.

  Note: The peak-width at base (W$_b$) may be called the "base width". However, the peak width at half height (W$_h$) must never be called the "half width" because that has a completely different meaning. Also, the symbol $w_{1/2}$ should never be used instead of W$_h$*

- ***Peak-Width at Inflection Points (W$_i$) (FG in Fig.2.2A and Fig. 2.4)***

  The length of the line drawn between the inflection points parallel to the peak base.

  In the case of Guassian (symmetrical) peaks, the peak-widths are related to the standard

  Deviation (σ) of the peak according to the following equations:

  $$w_b = 4\,\sigma$$

  $$w_i = 2\,\sigma$$

  $$w_h = 2\,\sigma\,\sqrt{4}\,(2\,\text{In}\,2) = 2.355\,\sigma$$

- ***Tailing***

  Asymmetry of a peak such that, relative to the baseline, the front is steeper than the rear. In paper chromatography and thin-layer chromatography, it refers to the distortion of a spot showing a diffuse region behind the spot in the direction of flow.

- ***Fronting***

  Asymmetry of a peak resulting due to overloading of the column and wherein the front part (start) of the peak is less steep than the rear. In paper chromatography and thin layer chromatography, it represents the distortion of the peak with diffused region in the 'front' of the spot in the direction of the flow. This contrasts with tailing where the diffusion of spot is 'behind' the direction of the flow.

- ***Step***

  The portion of an integral chromatogram recording the amount of a component, or the corresponding change in the signal from the detector as the component emerges from the column (see Fig. 2B).

- ***Step Height (NM in Fig. 2.2B)***

  The distance, measured in the direction of detector response, between straight-line extensions of the baselines on both sides of a step.

- ***Internal Standard***

  A compound added to a sample in known concentration to facilitate the qualitative identification and/or quantitative determination of the sample components.

- ***External Standard***

  A compound present in a standard sample of known concentration and volume which is analyzed separately from the unknown sample under identical conditions. It is used to facilitate the qualitative identification and/or quantitative determination of the sample components. The volume of the external standard (standard sample) need not to be known if it is identical to that of the unknown sample.

- ***Marker***

  A reference substance chromatographed with the sample to assist in identifying the components.

- ***Diffusion***

  The diffusion coefficient (D) is the amount of a particular substance that diffuses across a unit area in 1 s under the influence of a gradient of one unit.

  It is usually expressed in the units $cm^2 s^{-1}$.

- ***Diffusion Coefficient in the Stationary Phase (D_s or D_L)***

  The diffusion coefficient characterizing the diffusion in the stationary phase. In partition chromatography with a liquid stationary phase, the symbol D_L may be used to express this term.

- ***Diffusion Coefficient in the Mobile Phase (D_M or D_G)***

  The diffusion coefficient characterizing the diffusion in the mobile phase. In gas Chromatography where the mobile phase is a gas, the symbol D_G may be used to express this term.

- ***Diffusion Velocity (u_D)***

  This term is used in liquid chromatography in the expression of the reduced mobile-phase velocity. The diffusion velocity expresses the speed of diffusion into the pores of the particles:

$$u_D = D_M / d_p$$

Temperatures

- *Ambient Temperature (T_a)*

  The temperature outside the chromatographic system.

- *Injection Temperature (T_i)*

  The temperature within the injection device.

- *Separation Temperature (T_c)*

  The temperature of the chromatographic bed under isothermal operation. In column chromatography it is called the Column Temperature.

Temperatures during Programme Temperature Analysis

- *Initial Temperature*

  The temperature of the chromatographic bed (column) at the start of the analysis. Temperature programming might start immediately upon sample introduction or it can be preceded by a short isothermal period (Initial Isothermal Temperature). In this case, the time of the Initial Isothermal Period must also be specified.

- *Program Rate*

  The rate of increase of column temperature. The rate of temperature increase is usually linear ($^{\circ}$C/min) but it may also be non-linear. During one analysis the temperature rate may be changed and/or the temperature programming may be interrupted by an isothermal period. In this case one is speaking about Multiple Programming. In multiple programming each program must be specified by its initial and final temperatures and program rate.

- *Mid-Analysis Isothermal Temperature*

  The temperature of the column in an isothermal period during elution. The corresponding time (Mid-Analysis Isothermal Period) must also be specified.

- *Final Temperature*

  The highest temperature to which the column is programmed.

- *Final Isothermal Temperature*

  The final temperature of the program if it is followed by an isothermal period. The time corresponding to the Final Isothermal Period must also be specified.

- ***Retention Temperature***

  The column temperature corresponding to the peak maximum.

- ***Detector Temperature***

  The temperature of the detector cell. In the case of a detector incorporating a flame, it refers to the temperature of the detector base.

The Mobile Phase

- ***Mobile Phase Viscosity (η)***

  The viscosity of the mobile phase at the temperature of the chromatographic bed.

Pressures

- ***Inlet Pressure (p_i)***

  The absolute pressure at the inlet of a chromatographic column.

- ***Outlet Pressure (p_o)***

  The absolute pressure at the exit of a chromatographic column. It is usually but not necessarily equal to the Ambient Pressure (p_a), the atmospheric pressure outside the chromatographic system.

- ***Pressure Drop (Δp)***

  The difference between the inlet and outlet pressures: $\Delta p = p_i - p_o$

- ***Relative Pressure (P)***

  The ratio of the inlet and outlet pressures: $P = p_i / p_o$

- ***Mobile Phase Compressibility Correction Factor (j)***

  A factor, applying to a homogeneously filled column of uniform diameter, that corrects for the compressibility of the mobile phase in the column. It is also called the Compressibility.

- ***Correction Factor***

  In gas chromatography, the correction factor can be calculated as:

  $$j = \frac{3p^3 - 1}{2p^3 - 1} = \frac{3\,(pi/po)^2 - 1}{2(pi/po)^3 - 1}$$

  In liquid chromatography the compressibility of the mobile phase is negligible.

Note: In former nomenclatures the term "pressure gradient correction factor" was sometimes used to express the same term. This is, however, an incorrect name, because it is not the pressure gradient but the compression of the mobile phase which necessitates the use of this factor. In liquid chromatography, where mobile phase compression is negligible, no correction factor has to be applied to the mobile phase velocity; however, there is still a pressure gradient along the column.

- ***Flow Rate***

  The volume of mobile phase passing through the column in unit time.

  The flow rate is usually measured at column outlet, at ambient pressure (p_a) and temperature (T_a, in K); this value is indicated with the symbol F. If a water-containing flowmeter was used for the measurement (e.g., the so-called soap bubble flowmeter) then F must be corrected to dry gas conditions in order to obtain the Mobile Phase Flow Rate at Ambient Temperature (F_a):

  $$F_a = F \left(1 - p_w / p_a\right)$$

  Where p_w is the partial pressure of water vapor at ambient temperature.

  In order to specify chromatographic conditions in column chromatography, the flow-rate (Mobile Phase Flow Rate at Column Temperature, F_c) must be expressed at T_c (kelvin), the column temperature:

  $$F_c = F_a \left(T_c / T_a\right)$$

Velocities

- ***Mobile-Phase Velocity (u)***

  The linear velocity of the mobile phase across the average cross-section of the chromatographic bed or column. It can be calculated from the column flow-rate at column temperature (F_c), the cross-sectional area of the column (A_c) and the inter-particle porosity (ε):

  $$u = F_c / (\varepsilon A_c)$$

  In practice the mobile phase velocity is usually calculated by dividing the column length (L) by the retention time of an un-retained compound

  $$u = L / t_m$$

In gas chromatography, due to the compressibility of the carrier gas, the linear velocity will be different at different longitudinal positions in the column. Therefore two terms must be distinguished:

The Carrier Gas Velocity at Column Outlet (u_o) can be obtained as above, from the carrier gas flow rate measured at column outlet:

$$u_0 = F_c / (\varepsilon\, A_c)$$

The Average Linear Carrier Gas Velocity ($\bar{u}$) is obtained from u_o, by correcting it for gas compressibility:

$$\bar{u} = u_o j$$

The average linear carrier gas velocity can also be obtained by dividing column length (L) by there tention time of an un-retained compound (t_M):

$$\bar{u} = L / t_M$$

In liquid chromatography where mobile phase compression is negligible, $\bar{u} = u$

- ***Reduced Mobile Phase Velocity (u)***

  A term used mainly in liquid chromatography. It compares the mobile phase velocity with the velocity of diffusion into the pores of the particles (the so-called diffusion velocity, u_D:

  $$\upsilon = \bar{u} / u_D = \bar{u} d_p / D_M$$

  In open-tubular chromatography:

  $$\upsilon = \bar{u}\, d_c / D_M$$

Retention Parameters in Column Chromatography

Retention parameters may be measured in terms of chart distances or times, as well as mobile phase volumes; e.g., t_R' (time) is analogous to V_R' (volume). If recorder speed is constant, the chart distances are directly proportional to the times; similarly if the flow rate is constant, the volumes are directly proportional to the times.

- ***Hold-up Volume (Time) (V_M, t_M)***

  The volume of the mobile phase (or the corresponding time) required to elute a component the concentration of which in the stationary phase is negligible compared to that in the mobile phase. In other words, this component is not retained at all by the stationary phase. Thus, the hold-up volume (time) is equal to the *Retention Volume (Time) of an Unretained Compound.*

The hold-up volume (time) corresponds to the distance OA in Fig. 3A and it includes any volumes contributed by the sample injector, the detector, and connectors.

$$t_M = V_M / F_c$$

In gas chromatography this term is also called the *Gas Hold-up Volume (Time).*

- *Corrected Gas Hold-up Volume (V_M^o)*

The gas hold-up volume multiplied by the compression (compressibility) correction factor *(j)*:

$$V_M^o = V_M \cdot j$$

Assuming that the influence of extra column volume on V_M is negligible,

$$V_M^o = V_G$$

- *Total Retention Volume (Time) (V_R, t_R)*

The volume of mobile phase entering the column between sample injection and the emergence of the peak maximum of the sample component of interest (OB in Fig. 2.2A), or the corresponding time. It includes the hold-up volume (time):

$$t_R = V_R / F_c$$

- *Peak Elution Volume (Time)* $\left(\overline{V}_r, \overline{t}_r \right)$

The volume of mobile phase entering the column between the start of the elution and theemergence of the peak maximum, or the corresponding time. In most of the cases, this is equal to the total retention volume (time). There are, however, cases when the elution process does notstart immediately at sample introduction. For example, in liquid chromatography, sometimes the column is washed with a liquid after the application of the sample to displace certain components which are of no interest and during this treatment the sample does not move along the column. In gas chromatography, there are also cases when a liquid sample is applied to the top of the column but its elution starts only after a given period. This term is useful in such cases.

- *Adjusted Retention Volume (Time) (V_R', t_R')*

The total elution volume (time) minus the hold-up volume (time). It corresponds to the distance AB in Fig. 2A:

$$V'_R = V_R - V_M$$

$$t'_R = t_R - t_M = (V_R - V_M)/F_c = V'_R / F_c$$

- **Corrected Retention Volume (Time) (V_o^R, t_R^o)**

  The total retention volume (time) multiplied by the compression correction factor *(j)*:

  $$V_R^o = V_R\, j$$

  $$t_R^o = V'_R \cdot j / F_c = V_R^o / F_c$$

- **Net Retention Volume (Time) (V_N, t_N)**

  The adjusted retention volume (time) multiplied by the compression correction factor *(j)*:

  $$V_N = V'_R \cdot j$$

  $$t_N = V'_R \cdot j / F_c = V_N / F_c$$

  In liquid chromatography, the compression of the mobile phase is negligible and thus, the compression correction factor does not apply. For this reason, the total and corrected retention volumes (times) are identical $(V_R = V_R^o\,;\ t_R = t_N)$ and so are the adjusted and net retention volumes (times) $V'_R = V_N\,; t'_R = t_N$.

Specific Retention Volumes

- **The specific retention volume at column temperature $\left(V_g^\theta\right)$**

  The net retention volume per gram of stationary phase (stationary liquid, active solid or solvent free gel (W_s):

  $$V_g^\theta = V_N / W_s$$

- **Specific retention volume at 0^oC (V_g)**

  The value of V_g^θ corrected to $0°C$:

  $$V_g = V_g = \frac{\theta 273.15K}{T_c} = \frac{V_N}{W_S}\frac{273.15k}{T_c}$$

  Where T_c is the column temperature (in kelvin).

- ***Retention Factor (k)***

The retention factor is a measure of the time, the sample component resides in the stationary phase relative to the time it resides in the mobile phase: it expresses how much longer a sample component is retarded by the stationary phase than it would take to travel through the column with the velocity of the mobile phase. Mathematically, it is the ratio of the adjusted retention volume (time) and the hold-up volume (time):

$$k = V_R'/V_M = t_R'/t_M$$

If the distribution constant is independent of sample component concentration, then the retention factor is also equal to the ratio of the amounts of a sample component in the stationary and mobile phases respectively, at equilibrium:

$$K = \frac{amount\ of\ component\ in\ stationary\ phase}{amount\ of\ component\ in\ mobile\ phase}$$

If the fraction of the sample component in the mobile phase is R, then the fraction in the stationary phase is $(1 - R)$; thus

$$k = (1 - R)/R$$

- ***Logarithm of the Retention Factor***

This term is equivalent to the R, value used in planar chromatography. The symbol κ is suggested to express log k:

$$\kappa = \log k = \log [(1-R)/R]$$

- ***Retardation Factor (R)***

The fraction of the sample component in the mobile phase at equilibrium; it is related to the retention factor and other fundamental chromatography terms:

$$R = 1/(k+1)$$

Relative Retention Values

- ***Relative Retention (r)***

The ratio of the adjusted or net retention volume (time) or retention factor of a component relative to that of a standard, obtained under identical conditions:

$$r = V_{Ri}'/V_{R(st)}' = V_{Ni}/V_{N(st)} = t_{Ri}'/t_{R(st)}' = k_i/k_{st}$$

Depending on the relative position of the peak corresponding to the standard compound in the chromatogram, the value of r may be smaller, larger or identical to unity.

- ***Separation Factor (a)***

  The relative retention value calculated for two adjacent peaks

  $$\left(V'_{R2} > V'_{R1}\right) \alpha = V'_{R2}/V'_{R1} = V_{N2}/V_{N1} = t'_{R1} = k_2/k_1$$

  By definition, the value of the separation factor is always greater than unity. The separation factor is also identical to the ratio of the corresponding distribution constants.

  Note: The separation factor is sometimes also called the "selectivity". The use of this expression is discouraged.

- ***Unadjusted Relative Retention (r_G or α_G)***

  Relative retention calculated by using the total retention volumes (times) instead of the adjusted or net retention volumes (times):

  $$r_G = V_{Ri} / V_{R(st)} = t_{Ri}/ t_{R(st)} = \frac{k_1 + 1}{k_{st} + 1}$$

  subscript G commemorates E. Glueckauf, who first used this expression.

  Relative retention (r) and separation factor (α) values must always be measured under isothermal conditions. On the other hand, the 'unadjusted relative retention (r_G or α_G) values may also be obtained in programmed-temperature or gradient-elution conditions. Under such conditions, the symbol RRT (for Relative Retention Time) has also been used to describe the unadjusted relative retention values.

  Using the same stationary and mobile phases and temperature, the relative retention and separation factor values are reproducible between chromatographic systems. On the other hand, the unadjusted relative retention and ("relative retention time") values are only reproducible within a single chromatographic system.

- ***Retention Index; Kovats (Retention) Index (I)***

  The retention index of a sample component is a number, obtained by interpolation (usually logarithmic), relating the adjusted retention volume (time) or the retention factor of the sample component to the adjusted retention volumes (times) of two standards eluted before and after the peak of the sample component. In the Kovats Index or Kovats Retention Index used in gas chromatography, n-alkanes serve as the standards and logarithmic interpolation is utilized:

$$I = 100 \left[\frac{\log X_i - \log X_z}{\log X_{(z+1)} - \log X_z} + Z \right]$$

where X refers to the adjusted retention volumes or times, z is the number of carbon atoms of then-alkane eluting before, and (z + 1) is the number of carbon atoms of the n-alkane eluting afterthe peak of interest:

The Kovats (Retention) Index expresses the number of carbon atoms (multiplied by 100) of a hypothetical normal alkane which would have an adjusted retention volume (time) identical to that of the peak of interest when analyzed under identical conditions. The Kovats Retention Index is always measured under isothermal conditions. In the case of temperature-programmed gas chromatography a similar value can be calculated utilizing direct numbers instead of their logarithm. Since both the numerator and denominator contain the difference of two values, here we can use the total retention volumes (times). Sometimes this value is called the Linear Retention Index:

$$I^T = 100 \left[\frac{t^T_{Ri} - t^T_{Rz}}{t^T_{Rz+1} - t^T_{Rz}} \right] + Z$$

where t^T_R refers to the total retention times (chart distances) measured under the conditions of temperature programming. The value of I^T will usually differ from the value of I measured for the same compound under isothermal conditions, using the same two phases.

Retention Parameters in Planar Chromatography

- ### *Mobile-Phase Front*

  The leading edge of the mobile phase as it traverses the planar media. In all forms of development except radial, the mobile phase front is essentially a straight line parallel to the mobile phase surface. It is also called the Liquid Front or Solvent Front.

- *Mobile-Phase Distance*

  The distance travelled by the mobile phase travelling along the medium from the starting (application) front or line to the mobile phase front. It is the distance a in (Fig. 2.4).

- *Solute Distance*

  The distance travelled by the solute along the medium from the starting (application) point or line to the center of the solute spot. If the solute spot is not circular, an imaginary circle is used whose diameter is the smallest axis of the spot. It is the distance b in Fig. 2.4.

- *Retardation Factor (R_F)*

  Ratio of the distance travelled by the center of the spot to the distance simultaneously travelled by the mobile phase. Using the symbols of Fig. 2.4.

  $$R_F = b \, / \, a$$

  By definition the R_F, values are always less than unity. They are usually given to two decimal places. In order to simplify this presentation the hR_F, Values may be used: they correspond to the R_F values multiplied by 100.

  Ideally, the R_F, values are identical to the R values.

- *R_M Value*

  Alogarithmic function of the R_F, value:

  $$R_M = \log \frac{1 - RF}{RF} = \log \left[\frac{1}{RF} - 1 \right]$$

- *Relative Retardation (R_{rel})*

  This term is equivalent to relative retention used in column chromatography: it is the ratio of the R_F, value of a component to the R_F value of a standard (reference) substance. Since the mobile phase front is common for the two components, the R_{rel} value can be expressed directly as the ratio of the distances travelled by the spot of the compound of interest (b_i) and the reference substance (b_s) respectively:

  $$R_{rel} = R_{F(i)} \, / \, R_{F(st)} = b_i \, / \, b_{st}$$

  Note: In former nomenclatures the symbol Rs was used to express relative retardation in planar chromatography. Because of its identity with the symbol for peak resolution the symbol R_{rel} is suggested for relative retardation in planar chromatography.

Distribution Constants

The distribution constant is the concentration of a component in or on the stationary phase divided by the concentration of the component in the mobile phase. Since in chromatography a component may be present in more than one form (e.g., associated and dissociated forms), the analytical condition used here refers to the total amount present without regard to the existence of various forms.

These terms are also called the *Distribution Coefficients*. However, the present term conforms more closely to the general usage in science. The concentration in the mobile phase is always calculated per unit volume of the phase. Depending on the way the concentration in the stationary phase is expressed various forms of the distribution constants may exist.

- **Distribution Constant (K_c)**

  In the general case, the concentration in the stationary phase is expressed per unit volume of the phase. This term is mainly applicable to partition chromatography with a liquid stationary phase but can also be used with a solid stationary phase:

  Where $W_{i(s)}$ and $W_{j(M)}$ are the amounts of component 'i' in the stationary and mobile phases, while V_s and V_M are the volumes of the stationary and mobile phases, respectively.

  The term *Distribution Constant* and the symbol K_c, are recommended in preference to the term *Partition Coefficient* which has been in use in partition chromatography with a liquid stationary phase.

  The value of K_C, is related to the retention volume (V_R) of a sample component and the volumes of the stationary (V_s) and mobile phases (V_M) in the column:

  $$V_R = V_M + K_C V_S$$

  In gas chromatography both V_R and V_M have to be corrected for gas compressibility: therefore V_R° is to be used for V_R, and $V_G = V_M^\circ$ is to be used for V_M

  $$V_R^\circ = V_G + K_C \cdot V_S$$

- **Distribution Constant (K_g)**

  In the case of a solid stationary phase, the distribution constant may be expressed per *mass (weight) of the dry solid phase:*

$$K_g = \frac{W_t(s)/W_s}{W_t(M)/V_M}$$

where $W_{i(st)}$ and $W_{i(M)}$ are the amounts (masses) of the component 'i' in the stationary and mobile phases, respectively, W_{st}, is the mass (weight) of the *dry* stationary phase, and V_M is the volume of the mobile phase in the column.

- **Distribution Constant (K_s)**

  In the case of adsorption chromatography with a well characterized adsorbent of known surface area, the concentration in the stationary phase may be expressed per unit surface area:

$$K_s = \frac{W_i(s)/A_s}{W_t(M)/V_M}$$

- where $W_{i\,(s)}$ and $W_{i\,(M)}$ are the amounts (masses) of the component 'I' in the stationary and mobile phases, respectively, A_s, is the surface area of the stationary phase, and V_M is the volume of the mobile phase in the column.

Terms Expressing the Efficiency of Separation

- **Peak Resolution (R_s)**

  The separation of two peaks in terms of their average peak width at base ($t_{R2} > t_{R1}$):

$$R_s = \frac{(t_{R2} - t_{R1})}{(W_{b1} + W_{b2})/2} = \frac{2(t_{R2} - t_{R1})}{W_{b1} + W_{b2}}$$

  In the case of two adjacent peaks it may be assumed that $w_{bi} \approx w_{b2}$, and thus, the width of the second peak may be substituted for the average value:

$$R_s = (t_{R2} - t_{R1})/W_{b2}$$

- **Separation Number (SN)**

  This expresses the number of peaks which can be resolved in a given part of the chromatogram between the peaks of two consecutive n-alkanes with z and (z + 1) carbon atoms in their molecules:

$$SN = \frac{t_{R(z+1)} - t_{Rz}}{W_{hz} + W_{h(z+1)}} - 1$$

In the German literature the symbol TZ (Trennzahl) is commonly used to express the separation number.

As the separation number depends on the n-alkanes used for the calculation, they always must be specified with any given SN value.

- ***Plate Number (PN)***

A number indicative of column performance, calculated from the following equations which depend on the selection of the peak width expression:

$$N = (V_R / \sigma)^2 = (t_R/\sigma)^2$$
$$N = 16 (V_R /w_b)^2 = 16 (t_R/ w_b)^2$$
$$N = 5.545 (V_R/ w_h)^2 = 5.545 (t_R/ w_h)^2$$

The value of 5.545 stands for 8 ln 2. These expressions assume a Guassian (symmetrical) peak.

In these expressions the units for the quantities inside the brackets must be consistent so that their ratio is dimensionless: i.e., if the numerator is a volume, then peak width must also be expressed in terms of volume.

In former nomenclatures the expressions "Number of Theoretical Plates" or "Theoretical Plate Number" were used for the same term. For simplification, the present name is suggested.

- ***Effective Plate Number (N_{eff})***

A number indicative of column performance calculated by using the adjusted retention volume (time) instead of the total retention volume (time). It is also called the Number of Effective Plates:

$$N_{eff} = \left(V_R' /\sigma\right)^2 = \left(t_R' /\sigma\right)^2$$
$$N_{eff} = 16 (V_R' / w_b)^2 = 16 (t_R'/ w_b)^2$$
$$N_{eff} = 5.545 (V_R' / w_h)^2 = 5.545 (t_R'/ w_h)^2$$

The plate number and effective plate number are related to each other:

$$N = N_{eff} \left[\frac{k+1}{k}\right]^2$$

Where k is the retention factor.

- ***Plate Height (PH)***

The column length (L) divided by the plate number:

$$H = L / N$$

It is also called the Height Equivalent to One Theoretical Plate (HETP).

- ***Effective Plate Height (H_{eff})***

  The column length divided by the effective plate number:

  $$H_{eff} = L \, / \, N_{eff}$$

  It is also called the Height Equivalent to One Effective Plate.

- ***Reduced Plate Height (h)***

  A term used in liquid chromatography. It is the ratio of the plate height to the average particle diameter:

  $$H/dp \quad \text{For open-tubular columns:}$$
  $$h = H/dc$$

Terms Related to Detection and Classification of Detectors

Classification according to the Form of Response

- ***Differential Detector***

  These measure the instantaneous difference in the composition of the column effluent.

- ***Integral Detector***

  These measure the accumulated quantity of sample component(s) reaching the detector.

Classification according to the Basis of Response

- ***Concentration-Sensitive Detector***

  A device the response of which is proportional to the concentration of a sample component in the eluent.

- ***Mass-Flow Sensitive Detector***

  A device the response of which is proportional to the amount of sample component reaching thedetector in unit time.

Classification according to Detector Selectivity

- ***Universal Detector***

  A detector which responds to every component in the column effluent except the mobile phase.

- ***Selective Detector***
  A detector which responds to a related group of sample components in the column effluent.

- ***Specific Detector***
  A detector which responds to a single sample component or to a limited number of components having similar chemical characteristics.

Detector Response

The most significant detector requirement is its "sensitivity" as it defines the least concentration of solute that can be detected. It can be best explained as a function of the detector response and the noise level. The ***Detector Response*** can be defined as the voltage output from a detector that would result due to the unit change in solute concentration that is measured by the detector. ***Detector Noise*** can be defined as any interference on the detector output that is not associated to an eluted solute. It is a basic property of the detecting system and it determines the critical sensitivity or least amount of solute concentration that is detectable. Detector noise has been randomly divided into three types, ***'Short-term noise'***, ***'Long-term noise'*** and ***'Drift'*** as indicated in Fig.2.5.

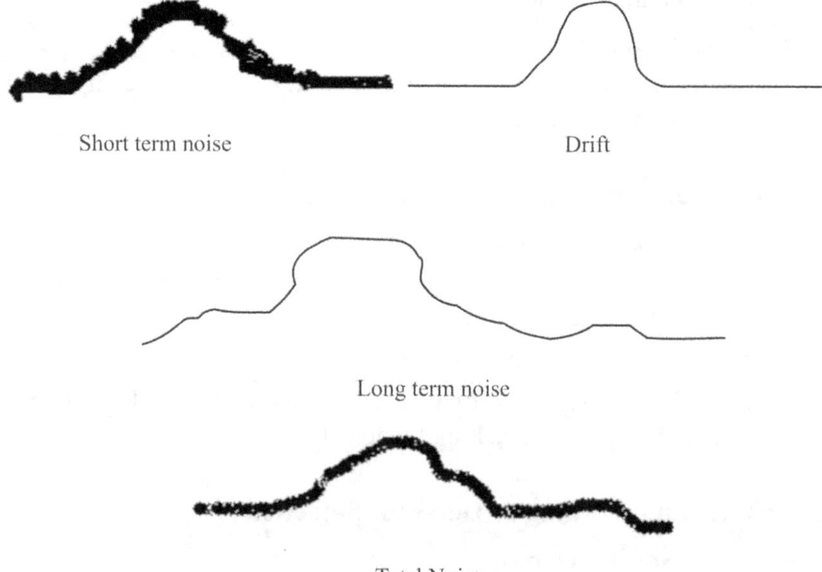

Figure 2.5 Different Types of Noise

Short-term noise consists of baseline perturbations that have a frequency that is considerably higher than the peak of the analyte. This type of noise can be easily removed by appropriate noise filters without considerably affecting the profiles of the peaks. The source of such short-term noise can be a electronic source like the detector sensor system or the amplifier.

Long-term noise comprise of baseline perturbations with a frequency similar to that of the eluted peak. This type of noise is of a major concern as it is barely visible from very small peaks in the chromatogram. Long-term noise *cannot* be eliminated by electronic filtering without disturbing the profiles of the eluted peaks. From Fig. 2.5, one can understand that the peak profile can easily be differentiated above the short term noise but is lost in the long-term noise. Long-term noise is usually a result of changes in temperature, pressure or flow rate of the sensing cell.

Drift is a baseline perturbation with a frequency larger than that of an eluted peak. Drift is mostly a result of the changes in ambient temperature, mobile flow rate, pressure changes, or changes in solvent composition. The detector noise is defined as the highest amplitude obtained as a result of the combined short– and long-term noise measured for a period of 15 minutes. The detector is connected to a column and mobile phase is passed through it for the measurement. The detector noise (ND) is calculated by constructing parallel lines that envelope the maximum amplitude of the recorder sketch over the defined time period as shown in Fig. 2.6.

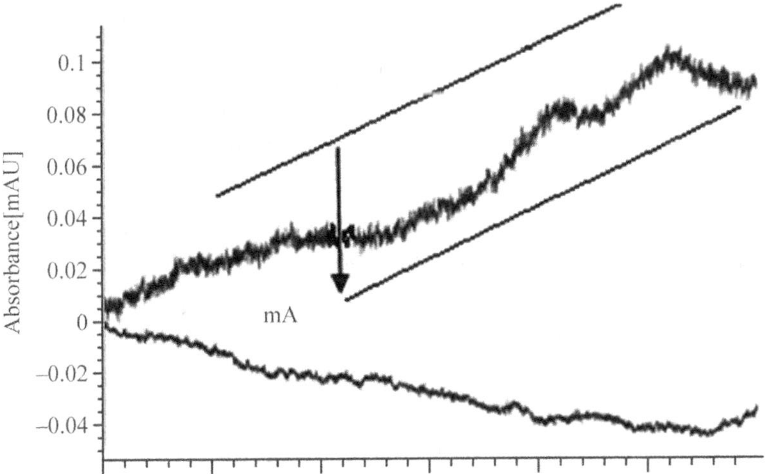

Figure 2.6 Measurement of detector noise

Detector sensitivity or minimum detectable concentration (MDC) is defined as the minimum concentration of solute passing through the detector that can be clearly distinguished from noise, usually considered when the signal to noise ratio is *two* and this principle has been adopted for estimating detector sensitivity. The two ranges that are specified for a detector are the *dynamic* range and the *linear dynamic* range (explained in further sections).

Detector Sensitivity (S)

The signal output per unit concentration or unit mass of a substance in the mobile phase entering the detector.

In the calculation of detector sensitivity the signal output of the detector is given as peak area in mV.min, A.s or AU.min (AU = absorbance unit). These values are obtained from the **integrated** peak area converted to the units specified.

Alternately, the peak area can also be obtained by multiplying the peak height at maximum (in mV, A or AU) by the peak-width at half height (in time units). The peak area calculated in this way will be 6% less than the true integrated peak area, assuming that the peak is Gaussian.

In the case of **concentration-sensitive detectors,** sensitivity is calculated per unit concentration in the mobile phase:

$$S = A_i F_c / W_i = E / C_i$$

where A_i is the integrated peak area (in mV.min or AU.min), E is the peak height (in mV or AU), C_i is the concentration of the particular substance in the mobile phase at the detector (ing.cm^{-3}), is the mobile phase flow rate corrected to column temperature (in cm^3.min^{-1}) and W is the mass (amount) of the substance present (in mg). The dimensions of detector sensitivity are mV.cm^3.mg^{-1} or AU.cm^3.mg^{-1}.

In the case of thermal-conductivity detectors, this sensitivity value is also called the **Dimbat-Porter-Stross Sensitivity** of the detector.

In the case of **mass-flow sensitive detectors,** sensitivity is calculated per unit mass of the test substance in the mobile phase entering the detector:

$$S = A_i / W_i = E_1 / M_j$$

Where A_i is the integrated peak area (in As), E is the peak height (in A), M_i is the mass rate of the test substance entering the detector (in g.s^{-1}), and W_i is the mass (amount) of test substance present (in g). The dimension of detector sensitivity is A.s.g^{-1} or C.g^{-1}.

Relative Detector Response Factor (f)

The relative detector response factor expresses the sensitivity of a detector relative to a standard substance. It can be expressed on an equal mole, equal volume or equal mass (weight) basis:

$$f_i = \left(A_i / A_{st} \right) f_{st}$$

where A refers to the peak area of the compound of interest (subscript i) and standard (subscript) respectively, and f_{st} is the response factor of the standard compound. Usually, an arbitrary value (e.g., 1 or 100) is assigned to f_{st}. Expressing the relative molar responses and using *n*-alkanes as the standards, the assigned value off, is usually the number of carbon atoms of the *n*-alkanes multiplied by 100 (e.g., 600 for n-hexane). If the relative detector response factor is expressed on an equal mass (weight) basis, the determined sensitivity values can be substituted for the peak area.

Noise and Drift

Noise (N) (see Fig. 2.7)

The amplitude expressed in volts, amperes, or absorbance units of the envelope of the baseline which includes all random variations of the detector signal the frequency of which is in the order of one or more cycles per minute. In the case of photometric detectors the amplitude may be expressed in absorbance units per unit cell length.

Drift (see Fig.2.7)

The average slope of the noise envelope, expressed in volts, amperes, or absorbance units per hour. It may be actually measured for 0.5 hour and extrapolated to one hour.

Minimum Detectability

The concentration or mass flow of a sample component in the mobile phase that gives a detector signal equal to twice the noise level. It can be calculated from the measured sensitivity (S) and noise (N):

$$D = 2N/S$$

where D is the minimum detectability, expressed either as concentration or mass-flow of thesubstance of interest in the mobile phase at the detector. Both sensitivity and minimumdetectability must be determined for the same substance.

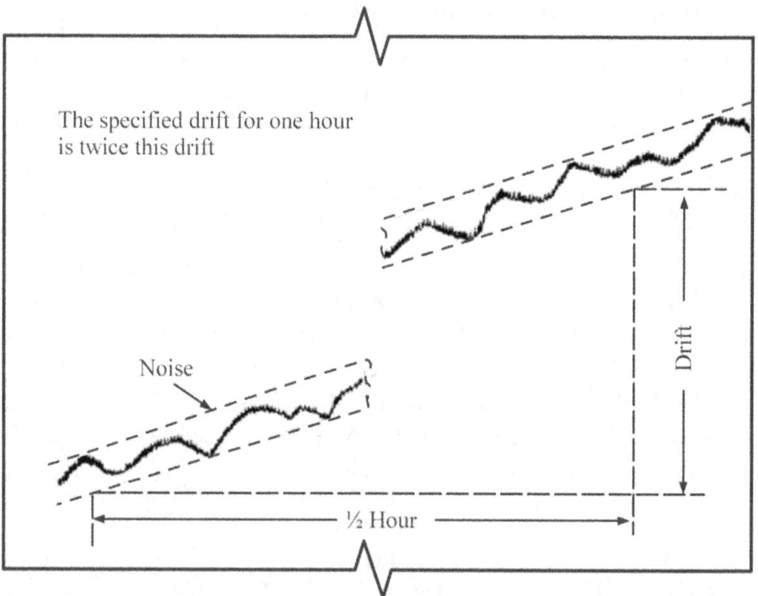

Figure 2.7 Measurement of the noise and drift of a chromatographic detector

Linear and Dynamic Ranges

- ***Linear Range***

  The linear range of a chromatographic detector represents the range of concentrations or mass flows of a substance in the mobile phase at the detector over which the sensitivity of the detector is constant within a specified variation, usually ± 5 percent. The best way to present detector linear range is the Linearity Plot (see Fig. 2.8) plotting detector sensitivity against amount injected, concentration or mass flow-rate. Here, the upper limit of linearity can be graphically established as the amount, concentration, or mass flow-rate) at which the deviation exceeds the specified value (± x% window around the plot). The lower limit of linearity is always the minimum detectable amount determined separately for the same compound.

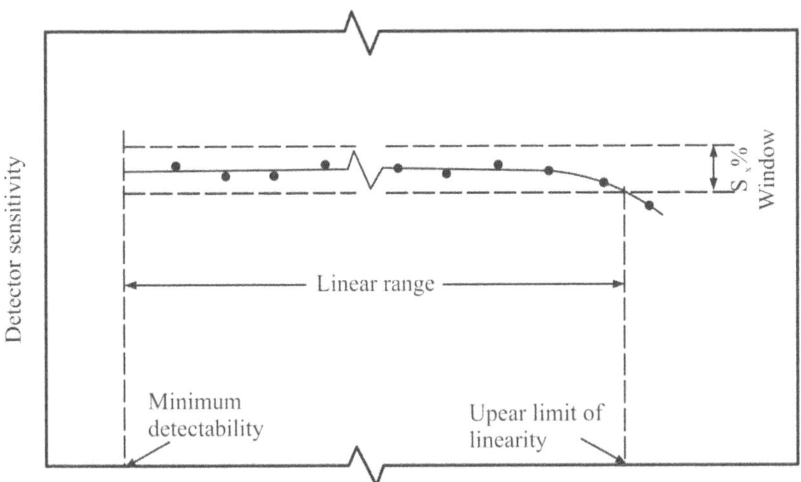

Figure 2.8 Linearity plot of a chromatographic detector. The scale of the ordinate is linear: the scale of the abscissa may be either linear or logarithmic

Alternatively, the linear range of a detector may be presented as the plot of peak area (height) against concentration or mass flow-rate of the test substance in the column effluent at the detector (see Fig. 2.9). This plot may be either linear or log/log. The upper limit of linearity is that concentration (mass flow-rate) at which the deviation from an ideal linearity plot is greater than the specified percentage deviation ($\pm$ x).

Numerically, the linear range can be expressed as the ratio of the upper limit of linearity obtained from the linearity plot and the minimum detectability, both measured for the same substance.

When presenting the linear range of a detector, either as a plot or as a numerical value, the test substance, the minimum detectability, and the specified deviation must be stated.

- ***Dynamic Range***

  The dynamic range of a detector is that range of concentration or mass flow-rates of a substance over which an incremental change in concentration or mass flow-rate produces an incremental change in detector signal. Fig. 2.9, presents a plot used for the determination of the dynamic range of a detector. The lower limit of the dynamic range is the minimum detectability. The upper limit is the highest concentration at which a further increase in concentration (mass flow-rate) will still give an observable increase in detector signal, and the dynamic range is the ratio of the upper and lower limits. The dynamic range is greater than the linear range. Numerically the dynamic range can be expressed as the ratio of the upper limit of the dynamic range obtained from the plot and the minimum detectability, both measured for the same substance.

When expressing the dynamic range of a detector, the test substance and the minimum detectability must be stated.

The Process of Chromatography

Chromatography is a process of separation of components of a mixture, which results due to the distribution of the individual components between stationary phase and the mobile phase. Those components which are held strongly in the stationary phase are retained for a longer time than those with a lower affinity. Thus, the solutes are eluted from the system in the order of their increasing distribution coefficients with respect to the stationary phase; and separation is achieved.

Whether the stationary phase is arranged in the form of a column or a plate, the mobile phase is allowed to pass through the stationary phase and elute the sample. The sample is introduced into the mobile phase flow just at the base of a plate or columns from where the mobile phase tends to carry the components based upon their relative affinities. The process can be represented as in Fig. 2.10.

Factors Controlling Retention

The Plate theory describes the equation for the retention volume (V_r), and is as follows:

$$V_r = V_m + KVS$$

Also, $$V_r' = KVS$$

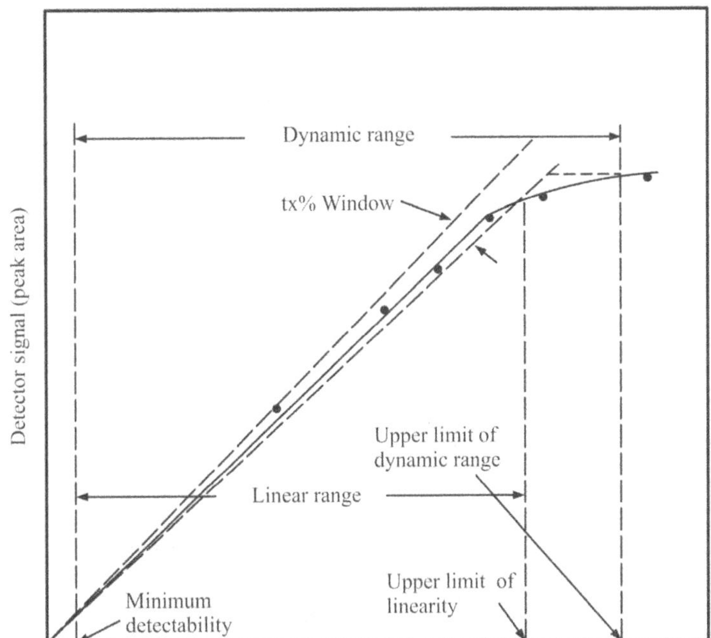

Figure 2.9 Determination of the linear and dynamic ranges of a chromatographic detector

Such a plot is usually in a log-log scale

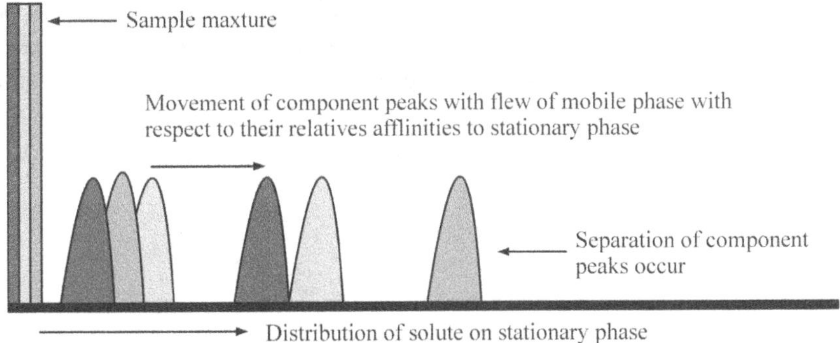

Figure 2.10 Separation of components in a chromatographic process

Thus, from the above equations it can be inferred that the corrected retention volume for a system are governed by two principal factors, viz. the *distribution coefficient of the solute between stationary phase and mobile phase.* Secondly, the *amount of stationary phase that is available for the solute.*

The Thermodynamic Processes in Retention

Classical thermodynamics provides an expression that explains the change in *free energy* of a solute components when being transferred from one phase to the other as a function of distribution coefficient. The expression is as follows,

$$RT \ln K = -\Delta G^o$$

where (R) is the gas constant, (G^o) is the Standard Free Energy Change and (T) is the absolute temperature.

Classical thermodynamics provides an additional expression for (ΔG^o), *i.e.*, where (ΔH^o) is the Standard Enthalpy Change, and (ΔS^o) is the Standard Entropy Change. Thus,

$$K = e - \frac{\Delta H_o}{RT} - \frac{\Delta S_o}{R}$$

$$\log K = \frac{\Delta H_o}{RT} + \frac{\Delta S_o}{R} \quad \text{and if,} \quad V' = KV_s$$

then
$$V' = -\frac{\Delta H_o}{RT} + \frac{\Delta S_o}{R} - \log V_s$$

It is observed that if the *standard entropy change* and *standard enthalpy change* for the distribution are calculated, then the distribution coefficient (K) and, the retention volume could also be estimated. Thus, a curve relating ln(V') and 1/T gives a straight line, of which slope will be proportional to the *standard enthalpy* and the intercept will be related to the *standard entropy*. Thus, the principal effects that control the distribution system can be recognized from such curves. Such curves are called Vant Hoff curves and an example of a Vant Hoff curve is given in Fig. 2.11.

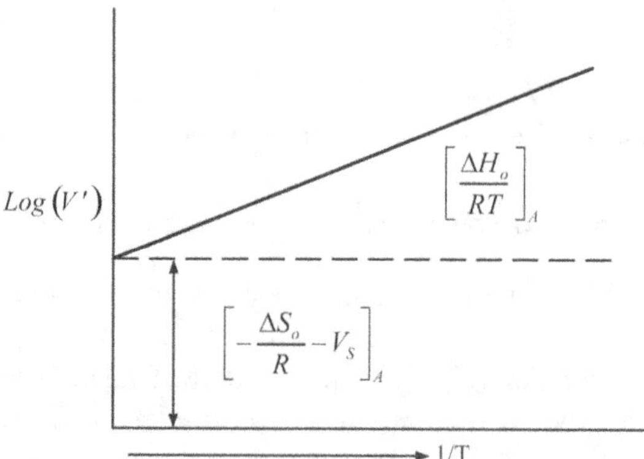

Figure 2.11 A representative Vant Hoff curve in a chromatographic process

Factors affecting the Magnitude of the Distribution Coefficient (K)

The magnitude of (K) is based upon the relative affinity of the solute with the stationary phase and the mobile phase. Those solutes which interact more strongly with the stationary phase have a larger distribution coefficient and will be retained longer in the chromatographic system. Molecular interaction results from intermolecular forces which are of three basic types: *dispersion forces*, *polar forces* and *ionic forces*.

- ***Dispersion Forces***

  Dispersion forces can be best explained considering the example of a molecule with various arrangements of nuclei and electrons having dipole moments. If the varying dipoles are averaged for a large number of configurations the resultant dipole would be zero. However, if there is any electrical interaction with other molecule interactive forces would be formed.

  Dispersive interactions are the result of many fluctuating closely associated charges (and not a particular localized part of a molecule) that can interact with charges of an opposite kind situated in a neighbouring molecule (see Fig. 2.12).

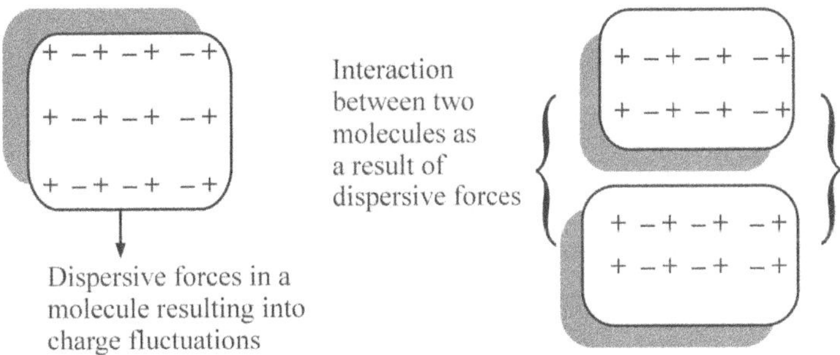

Figure 2.12 Interactive dispersion forces in molecules

- ***Polar Forces***

  Polar interactions are a result of the electrical forces between localized charges from permanent or induced dipoles. Examples of such occurrence are 'hydrogen bonding' as that of water with itself (Fig. 2.13). The molecules of water associate strongly with each other and also with the molecules of other polar solvents. Polar forces are accompanied by dispersive interactions and are sometimes also combined with ionic interactions.

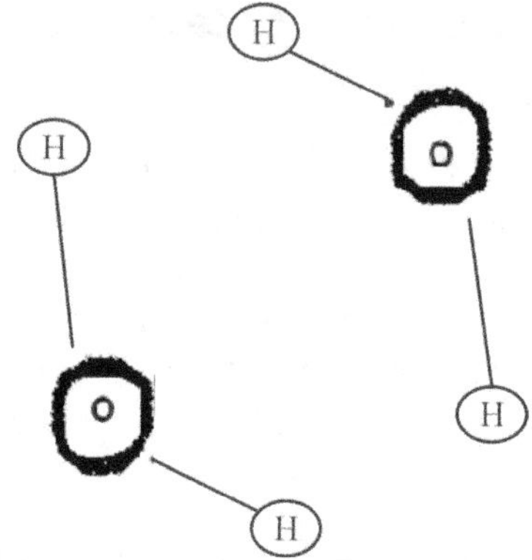

Figure 2.13 Polar interactions of water molecules with each other

- ***Ionic Forces***

  Polar compounds with dipoles do not have any net charge. However, ions possess a net charge and as a result can interact strongly with ions having an opposite charge. Ionic interactions are used to benefit in ion exchange chromatography where the counter ions to the ions being separated are located in the stationary phase.

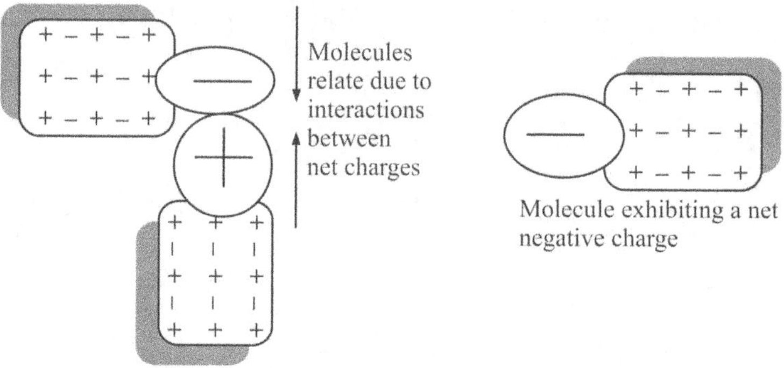

Figure 2.14 Ionic interactions of molecules with opposite charges

Hydrophobic and Hydrophilic Interactions of Solvents

The term "***hydrophobic interaction***" describes some form of molecular repulsion, or in other words a *dispersive* force towards water. The term can be best illustrated with the example of the immiscibility of a dispersive solvent such as *n*-heptane with a polar solvent like water. The term "hydrophilic interactions", literally means affinity for water. It corresponds to the term polar in case of interactions in a chromatographic method. Polar solvents are hydrophilic in nature due to their strong interactions with other solvents that arc polar in nature.

The Control of Chromatographically Available Stationary Phase (V_s)

The dimensions of stationary phase available to the solutes can be controlled through a number of ways. One of the ways is to vary the loading of sample on the stationary phase and adjusting the retention as required. A *particular* stationary phase loading may be selected, to either get better resolution, or to decrease the analysis time, or in some cases, to enhance the *sample* load. Sometimes, the stationary phase loading is reduced so the column is more amenable to specific compounds (e.g. to prevent proteins from being denatured). Secondly, the stationary phase can be made up of molecules of a particular shape that can only make *close* contact with solute molecules having a corresponding shape. Other molecules, which have differences in size will be unable to make close contact with the stationary phase and thus the stationary phase available to them will be restricted. This phenomenon is applied in chiral chromatography where the stationary phase is made up of a considerable proportion of largely of a specific enantiomer that gives chiral selectivity to system. Also, the stationary phase can be linked to the surface of a porous support, and the size of the analyte molecules to be separated will depend upon the pore size of the support on stationary phase. In such conditions, the larger molecules will be removed from the pores and smaller particles will be entrapped in the stationary phase bed. Thus, much less of the stationary phase will be available for larger molecules. This phenomenon is utilized in size exclusion chromatography (SEC) where analytes are separated on the basis of molecular size.

The Effect of Stationary Phase Loading on the Performance of a Chromatographic System

Separation is affected by two ways by the stationary phase material of a column. The greater the volume of stationary phase in a column, the more the solutes will be retained; the better will be the separation. Any change in stationary phase, conversely, changes the retention of all solutes proportionally and, thus, the separation increases, only if the *peak widths* remain unchanged. Increase in the amount of stationary phase generally increases the thickness of the stationary phase layer, and peak dispersion is increased. Basically, a specific amount for stationary phase loading should be arrived upon that provides the best compromise between separation and band dispersion thus, providing the highest resolution.

The Theoretical Plate Model of Chromatography

The first and most vital characteristic of chromatography theory that needs to be primarily understood is the Plate Theory.

- ***The Plate Theory***

  The plate theory states that the solute, while passing through the column, is always in equilibrium with the mobile phase and stationary phases. However, equilibrium between the phases *never* occurs in reality. While assuming the non-equilibrium condition, the column is considered to be divided into a number of theoretical plates.

  Equilibrations of the sample solute between the stationary and mobile phase occur in these "theoretical plates" independently. The sample solute moves down the column by transport of equilibrated mobile phase from one plate to the next.

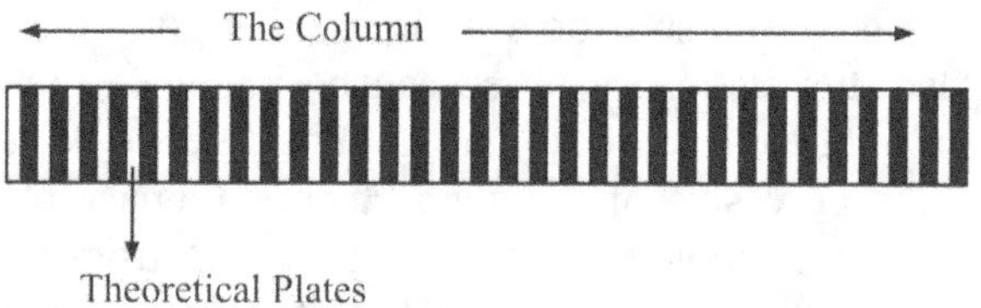

Figure 2.15 Theoretical plates in a column considered by plate theory

  However, one must remember that the plates do not really exist; they are a fabrication of the imagination that helps us understand the progressions in the column. They also serve as a method of estimating column efficiency, either by stating the number of theoretical plates in a column, N, or the plate height; the Height Equivalent to a Theoretical Plate (HETP).

  If the length of the column is L, then the HETP can be calculated as:

  $$HETP = L/N$$

  The number of theoretical plates that a real column has can be found by examining a chromatographic peak after being eluted by the following equation;

$$N = \frac{5.55tR^2}{w_{1/2}^2}$$

where $w_{1/2}$ is the peak width at half-height and t_R is the retention time.

- ***The Rate Theory of Chromatography***

  A more realistic approach towards the processes that take place inside a column considers the time taken for the solute to equilibrate between the stationary and mobile phase. This is in contrast to the plate model, which assumes that equilibration is infinitely fast. The shape of a chromatographic peak in the system is affected by the rate of elution. It is also affected by the different paths that the solute molecule travels between particles of stationary phase. Van Deemter and coworkers assumed that there were four processes that resulted into peak dispersion, viz., *multi-path dispersion, longitudinal diffusion, resistance to mass transfer in the mobile phase* and *resistance to mass transfer in the stationary phase.* Considering the various mechanisms which contribute to band broadening, **Van Deemter** derived an equation for plate height;

  $$HETP = A + B/u + Cu$$

  where u is the average velocity of the mobile phase. A, B, and C are the factors which contribute to band broadening.

- ***Van Deemter Plot***

  A Van Deemter plot is a plot of plate height vs. average linear velocity of mobile phase and are considered for determining the optimum mobile phase flow rate.

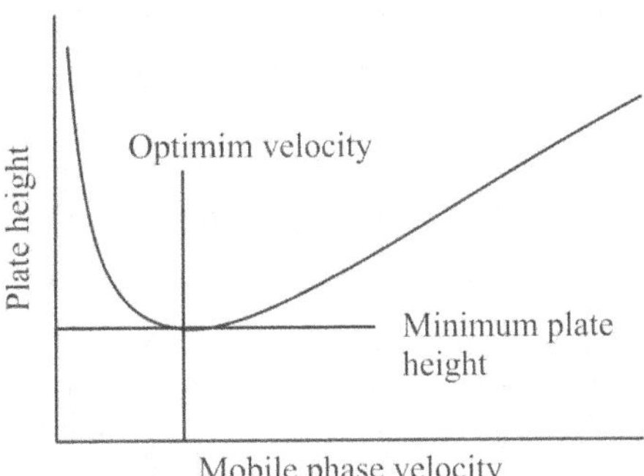

Figure 2.16 A typical Van Deemeter plot

- *A - Eddy Diffusion*

  The mobile phase moves through the stationary phase in a tortuous path in between the interstices of the particles with results in formation of eddies, like that of the obstructions to the flow of water by pebbles or stones in the path. The solute molecules will randomly take different paths for movement through the stationary bed. Some particles will take shorter routes and move faster, whereas some may take longer paths and have a slow movement. These different paths are of different lengths and cause a difference in the distances travelled by different molecules and results in band broadening.

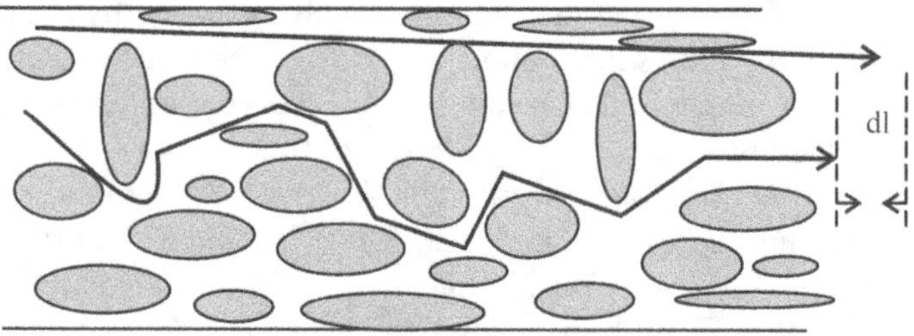

Figure 2.17 Multiple path movement (eddy diffusion)

- *B - Longitudinal Diffusion*

  The concentration of analyte is more around the centre of the band as compared to the edges. Due to the movement of the mobile phase the dispersion of solute molecules occur and separation of components occurs. As the mobile phase causes diffusion of analyte diffuses out from the center to the edges. This causes band broadening. When the velocity of the mobile phase increases, then the solute molecules have very less time to be spent in the column, this decreases the effects of longitudinal diffusion.

- *C - Resistance to Mass Transfer in the Mobile Phase*

  When the mobile phase moves through the column it carries along with it, the particles of the solute. Along with the movement of mobile phase the solute molecules slowly are transferred to the stationary phase in a reversible manner. The analyte molecules enter the stationary phase through an interface in a slow and gradual manner by diffusion. Only those particles which enter the stationary phase remain adhered to it, and rest of the molecules are carried away along with the continuous flow of the mobile phase. The rest of the particles that are carried away by the mobile phase travel further and undergo the same process as that of the previous component that had entered the stationary phase interface initially. This is how the transfer of analyte occurs in and out of the stationary phase. Faster is the interaction of solute and stationary phase smaller is the transfer of solute mass into the stationary phase. Faster the movement of mobile phase, lesser is the analyte and stationary phase interaction and lesser is the mass transfer.

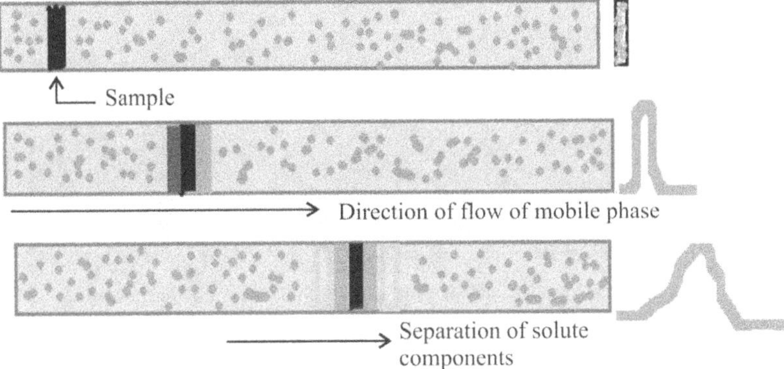

Figure 2.18 Longitudinal diffusion of band by mobile phase

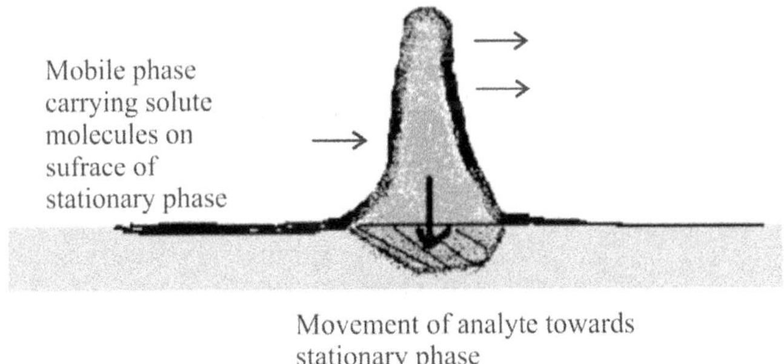

Figure 2.19 Transfer of solute between phases

Freundlich Adsorption Isotherm

The Freundlich adsorption isotherm, is a curve that relates the concentration of a analyte on the surface of an stationary phase, to the concentration of the analyte in the mobile phase with which it is in contact. In the year 1909, Freundlich gave an empirical expression that represented the isothermal variation of adsorption of an amount of gas adsorbed by unit mass of solid adsorbent under pressure. This equation is known as *Freundlich Adsorption Isotherm* or *Freundlich Adsorption equation.*

There are fundamentally two well recognized types of adsorption isotherms: the Freundlich adsorption isotherm and the Langmuir adsorption isotherm.

Freundlich adsorption isotherm

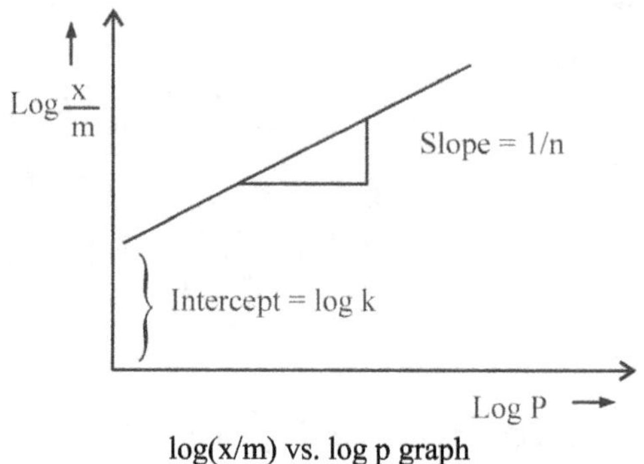

log(x/m) vs. log p graph

Figure 2.20 A typical Freundlich Adsorption Isotherm

The Freundlich Adsorption Isotherm is mathematically expressed as

$$x/m = Kp^{1/n}$$

It is also written as

$$\log(x/m) = \log k + (1/n)\log p$$

Also as, $x/m = Kp^{1/n}$

or also as $\log(x/m) = \log k + (1/n)\log c$

Where, x = mass of adsorbate

m = mass of adsorbent

p = Equilibrium pressure of adsorbate

c = Equilibrium concentration of adsorbate in solution.

K and n are constants for a given adsorbate and adsorbent at a particular temperature.

At high pressure $1/n = 0$

Thus, the extent of adsorption is independent of pressure. But at high pressure it is dependent on pressure.

- ***Limitations of Freundlich Adsorption Isotherm***

  Through various experiments it was determined that extent of adsorption varies directly with pressure till saturation pressure P_s is reached. Beyond that point rate of adsorption saturates even after a higher pressure is applied. Thus, Freundlich Adsorption Isotherm demonstrates a failure at higher pressure.

Langmuir Adsorption Isotherm

In the Langmuir adsorption isotherm the amount of mass that is adsorbed is plotted against the temperature and it explains the variation of adsorption with temperature.

Langmuir proposed his theory based upon the following assumptions:

(i) A fixed number of adsorption sites are available on the surface of solid adsorbent.

(ii) All the adsorption sites are of equal size and shape on the surface of adsorbent.

(iii) And, each site can hold maximum of one gaseous molecule and a constant amount of heat energy is released during this course.

(iv) A dynamic equilibrium is present between adsorbed gaseous molecules and the free gaseous molecules.

$$A(g) + B(S) \underset{\text{desorption}}{\overset{\text{Adsorption}}{\rightleftharpoons}} AB$$

Where A (g) is un-adsorbed gaseous molecule, B(s) is unoccupied metal surface and AB is Adsorbed gaseous molecule.

(v) Adsorption is of a monolayer type.

The Langmuir Equation was derived by introduction of the parameter 'θ'. Where 'θ' was considered as the number of sites of the surface which are covered with gaseous molecules. Thus, the fraction of surface which are not covered by gaseous molecules will be $(1 - \theta)$.

As, the rate of forward direction depends upon number of sites available on the surface of adsorbent, $(1 - \theta)$ and Pressure, P, and the rate of reaction is directly proportional to both mentioned factors, one arrives to the derivation:

$$\text{Rate of forward reaction} \propto P(1 - \theta)$$

$$\text{Rate of adsorption} \propto P(1 - \theta)$$

or $\qquad \text{Rate of adsorption} = K_a P(1 - \theta)$

Similarly, Rate of Desorption is dependent upon number of sites occupied by the gaseous molecules on the surface of adsorbent. Thus,

$$\text{Rate of desoption} \; \alpha \; \theta$$

or, $\qquad \text{Rate of desorption} = K_d \, \theta$

At equilibrium, rate of adsorption is equal to rate of desorption which concludes as :

$$K_a P(1 - \theta) = K_d \, \theta$$

- ***Limitations of Langmuir Adsorption Equation***

Based upon the various experiments carried out to determine the validity of the isotherm theory, it was found that **Langmuir equation is valid only under low pressure conditions,** which is a limitation to the Adsorption Equation.

Plumber's View of Chromatography

Plumber's view theory states that every analyte has a particular capacity factor (k') that describes the amount of time an analyte spends in the stationary phase and with the mobile phase.

i.e., $\qquad k' = \dfrac{t_r - t_M}{t_M} = \dfrac{V_s}{V_m}$

It explains that analytes with different partition coefficients will exhibit different retention times. A chromatography depends on the retention time, and it is demonstrated that the mobile phase will be always move faster than an analyte. This is because there is a minimum of interaction between the sorbent (stationary phase) and the solvent system (mobile phase).

If "q" is fraction of solute in mobile phase, then

$$q = \frac{moles_m}{moles_m + moles_s}$$

$$q = \frac{1}{1 + \dfrac{C_s V_s}{C_m V_m}} = \frac{1}{+k\dfrac{V_s}{V_m}}$$

thus, $\qquad q = \dfrac{1}{1 + k'}$ (i.e, the fraction in MP)

and

$$(1 - q) = \frac{k'}{1 + k'} \quad \text{(i.e., the fraction in SP)}$$

Solvent Selection for a Chromatography Method

- *Snyder's Triangle Method*

   In 1970s, Rohrschneider studied the properties of various solvents and showed that, in some cases, when two solvents were mixed, properties of a third solvent could be obtained. This recommended that some subset of most of the solvents could possibly be used for chemical purposes. During the same period, Lloyd Snyder worked upon various solvent properties that were important in chromatographic separations, especially reversed-phase liquid chromatography. From supplementary studies, he knew that three properties were of particular importance as far as the issue of selectivity is concerned. They are the properties of the acidic, basic and dipolar nature of the solvents. Snyder recalculated Rohrs-chneider's data based on these three properties and plotted them as solvent selectivity triangle. A subset of these data is shown in Fig. 2.21, where each solvent is plotted according to its proportion of acidic, basic and dipolar properties. The heavy dots indicate the central tendency of several solvent classes, some of which are labeled.

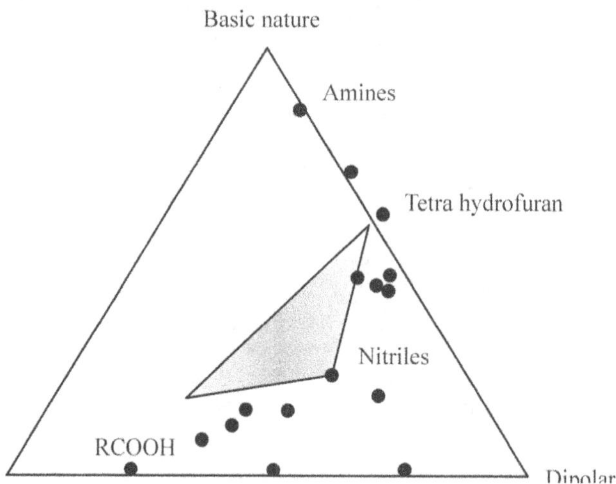

Figure 2.21 Solvent selection triangle

In principle, three solvents one with 100% acidity, one with 100% basicity and one with 100% dipolarity are assumed to be located at the extreme corners of the triangle. If these solvents existed, one should be able to combine them in varying proportions and obtain the properties of solvents lying within the boundaries of the triangle. Although such solvents do not exist, most of the solvents have a mixture of acidic, basic and dipolar properties, so they fall in the region away from the corner and usually away from the edges of the triangle. As the preferred solvents do not exist at the corners of the triangle, one would consider other solvents that are close to the corners solvents that exhibit primarily acidic, basic or dipolar properties. For example, carboxylic acids (RCOOH in Fig. 2.21) are quite acidic, amines (like triethylamine) are basic, and chlorinated solvents (like dichloromethane, $MeCl_2$) have dipole properties. If these three solvents are blended together, one might expect to get intermediate properties. But however, since the chlorinated solvents don't mix with the others and two phases result in an undesirable mobile phase characteristic for a analyst. One can continue working in the path towards the center of the triangle, searching for solvents that are miscible and have an influence of one of the desired properties. Alcohols have some acidic properties, ethers have basic properties, and nitriles have dipole properties. Such types of solvents are mutually miscible and form a subset (shaded area) of the total triangle.

This solvent triangle approach of development of method was very popular in the 1970s and 1980s. It was reasonably insightful to use and it generated useful methods. It was equally good for developing isocratic and gradient methods. However, because the mobile phases were often composed of all three solvents plus water, they were complex and were less reproducible.

- ***Hildebrand Solvent Scale***

The Hildebrand solvent scale is a list of general solvents used in Liquid Chromatography in order of their increasing energies of adsorption on alumina. The values differ from the values on silica gel or alumina, but the order is essentially the same. (see Hildebrand solubility values in **Appendix 1**)

- ***Selection of Starting Solvent***

The starting solvent for a given separation can be selected by corresponding the relative polarity of the solvent to that of the sample. This is done initially as an approximation by selecting the solvent to match the most polar functional group on the selected analyte (e.g. alcohols for OH, amines for NH_2, etc.). Then, the separation process can be improved by the following procedure:

If the sample appears at the solvent front then the solvent is too polar to allow the adsorbent to slow down the sample. A solvent of lower polarity on the scale should be selected.

On the other hand if the sample does not appear in a considerable time one should switch to a solvent of higher polarity on the scale.

A list of elutropic series is given in Table 2.1. The general separation problems can be overcomed by changing the solvent strength, column temperature or pH of mobile phase. While changing the solvent in isocratic runs, the modifier concentration can be increased or decreased with a few per cent. In gradient runs, the gradient steepness can be changed. While attempting for change of column temperature, the temperature change should be $\pm10°C$. The pH of the mobile phase should be changed by ±0.5 pH units.

However, chromatographic method for any substance, would exhibit various problems depending upon various chromatographic parameters which affect separation and resolution, systematic (determinate), operational and personal errors.

TABLE 2.1

Elutropic series of solvents in chromatography

Solvent	ε° Al_2O_3	ε° SiOH	ε° C_{18}	P'
Pentane	0.00	0.00	-	0
Hexane	0.00-0.01	0.00-0.01	-	0.1
Iso-octane	0.01	0.01	-	0.1
Cyclohexane	0.04	0.03	-	0.2
Carbon tetrachloride	0.17-0.18	0.11	-	1.6
l-Chlorobutane	0.26-0.30	0.2	-	1
Xylene	0.26	-	-	2.5
Toluene	0.20-0.30	0.22	-	2.4
Chlorobenzene	0.30-0.31	0.23	-	2.7
Benzene	0.32	0.25	-	—
Ethyl ether	0.38	0.38-0.43	-	2.8
Dichloromethane	0.36-0.42	0.32-0.32	-	3.1
Chloroform	0.36-0.40	0.26	-	4.1
1,2-Dichloroethane	0.44-0.49	-	-	3.5
Methyl ethyl ketone	0.51	-	-	5.7
Acetone	0.56-0.58	0.47-0.53	8.8	5.1
Dioxane	0.56-0.61	0.49-0.51	11.7	4.8
1-Pentanol	0.61	-	-	-
Tetrahydrofuran	0.45-0.62	0.53	3.7	4
Methyl t-butyl ether	0.3-0.62	0.48	-	2.5
Ethyl acetate	0.58-0.62	0.38-0.48	-	4.4
Dimethyl sulfoxide	0.62-0.75	-	-	7.2
Diethylamine	0.63	-	-	-
Acetonitrile	0.52-0.65	0.50-0.52	3.1	5.8
1-Butanol	0.7	-	-	3.9
Pyridine	0.71	-	-	5.3
2-Methoxyethanol	0.74	-	-	5.5
n-Propyl alcohol	0.78-0.82	-	10.1	4
Isopropyl alcohol	0.78-0.82	0.6	8.3	3.9
Ethanol	0.88	-	3.1	-
Methanol	0.95	0.70-0.73	1.0	5.1
Ethylene glycol	1.11	-	-	-
Dimethyl formamide	-	-	7.6	6.4
Water	-	-	-	10.2

Note: ε° - is the measure of relative elution strength.

The expected order of elution for of compounds of organic classes would be as follows:

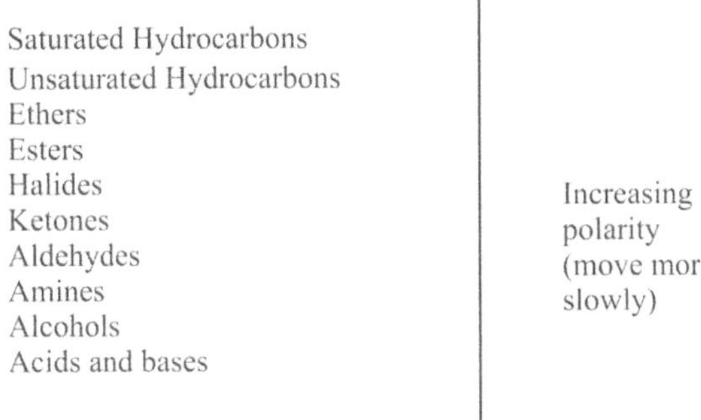

And the eluting power of organic solvents would be as follows:

Quantitative Analysis

In quantitative analysis, object is to resolve the exact number of analyte molecules in the sample. Most often two different analytes of equal concentration give varying detector responses in chromatography; thus detector responses should be recorded for identified concentrations of each analyte. A calibration analysis curve shows the detector response as a function of analyte concentration in the sample. For quantification analysis, three methods of calibration analysis are common:

    (i) *External standard calibration*

    (ii) *Internal standard calibration*

    (iii) *Standard addition method*

The ***External Standard Calibration Method*** is simple but less specific method and is generally used only when sample preparation is uncomplicated and small and no instrumental variations are observed. The method is not appropriate for use with complicated matrices. The term ***"External Standard Calibration"*** means that the standards are analyzed in chromatographic runs that are separate from those of unknown samples.

The ***Internal Standard (I. S.) Method*** is a more precise method than the other two methods. The I.S. method can balance for both instrument and sample preparation errors and variations (e.g. dilution and extraction). Sample pre-treatment steps such as extraction often lead to sample losses and a suitable I.S should be selected to imitate the variations in these steps. Thus both the precision and accuracy of quantitative data are enhanced if an I.S. is included in the procedure. The I.S. must be similar but not identical to the analyte, and both the internal standard and the analyte should be well resolved in the chromatographic step. The standard curves are obtained from standards of blank samples spiked with various known concentrations of the analyte of interest and adding up of an I.S. at constant concentration. Also the same constant concentration of I.S. should be added to the unknown samples. The unknown samples and the standard samples are processed in parallel with each other. In calibration curve the ratio of analyte to the I.S. peak area (or height) are plotted versus the analyte concentration.

An I.S. in a chromatographic method should fulfill the following criteria:

- Should be well resolved from the peak of the compound of interest and other peaks
- Have similar retention to the analyte
- It should not be present as a component in the sample
- Should be stable in nature
- Have a high purity (should not be contaminated with the analyte)
- Should resemble the analyte in all sample preparation steps
- Be of almost similar structure as of analyte
- Be of similar concentration as that of analyte

Most of the times a compound with a similar structure is selected as an I.S. The internal standard method has been accepted not only in chromatography, but is also popular in quantitative HPLC methods. The standard addition method is used often when it is not possible to obtain suitable blank matrices. The method involves addition of different weights of analyte to the unknown sample, which initially contains an unknown concentration of analyte. After the chromatographic run the peak areas (or heights) are plotted versus the added concentration. Extrapolation of the calibration plot provides the actual unknown concentration of analyte.

The ***Standard Addition Method*** involves injection of a sample with unknown concentration. A known amount of the substance which should be analyzed is added and analysis is performed after each addition. The unknown concentration is calculated by setting the value of Y = 0 in concentration response curve.

Appendix 1 Hildebrand Solvent Scale

Solvent	ri	UV cutoff	Viscosity (cP) at 20°C	Hildebrand solubility parameter	E° SiO_2	E° Al_2O_3	polarity index (Snyder)	BP (°C)
acetaldehyde diethyl acetal	1.379							
acetic acid	1.372	210	1.1-1.26	12.4		large	6.2	117.9
acetic anhydride	1.389							
Acetone	1.359	330	0.32	9.6	0.47-0.53	0.56-0.58	5.4	56.3
Acetonitrile	1.344	190	0.37	11.7	0.5	0.55-0.65	6.2	81.6
Benzene	1.501	280	0.65	9.2	0.25	0.32	3	80.1
Benzonitrile			1.22				4.6	191.1
benzyl alcohol			5.8				5.5	205.5
benzyl ether			5.33				3.3	288.3
butanol, 1-							3.9	117.2
butanol, 2-	1.395							
butanone, 2-	1.377							
butyl acetate	1.392							
butyl acetate, sec-	1.387							
butyl ether			0.7				1.7	142.2
butyl ethyl ether	1.380							
butyl formate	1.387							
butylamine, 2-	1.390							
Butyraldehyde	1.378							

Appendix 1 *contd…*

72

Solvent	ri	UV cutoff	Viscosity (cP) at 20°C	Hildebrand solubility parameter	E° SiO_2	E° Al_2O_3	polarity index (Snyder)	BP (°C)
butyric acid	1.396							
Butyronitrile	1.382							
carbon tetrachloride	1.466	265	0.97	8.6	0.12	0.18	1.7	76.5
chlorobutane, 2-	1.395							
Chloroform	1.443	245	0.57	9.2	0.26	0.36-0.4	3.4-4.4	61.2
chloropropane, 1-	1.386							
chloropropane, 2-	1.376							
Cyclohexane	1.427	200	0.98	8.2	0.04	0.04	0	80.7
cyclohexanone			2.24				4.5	155.7
dichloroethane							3.7	83.4
dichloromethane	1.424	232	0.44	9.6	0.32	0.4	3.4	40
diethyl carbonate	1.385							
di-isopropylamine	1.390							
dimethyl formamide, N,N-	1.431	268	0.90-0.92	11.5			6.4	153
dimethyl sulfoxide	1.478		2.24	12.8	0.41	0.62	6.5	189
dimethylbutane, 2,2-	1.369							
dimethylbutane, 2,3-	1.372							
dimethylpentane, 2,3-	1.389							
dimethylpentane, 2,4-	1.379							

Appendix 1 *contd...*

Solvent	ri	UV cutoff	Viscosity (cP) at 20°C	Hildebrand solubility parameter	$E°$ SiO_2	$E°$ Al_2O_3	polarity index (Snyder)	BP (°C)
dioxane, 1,4-							4.8	101
dioxane, p			1.54				4.8	101.3
dodecafluoro-1-hepatanol	1.316							
ethanol	1.361	205-210	1.2	12	0.68	0.88	5.2	78.3
ethyl acetate	1.370	256	0.46-0.47	9.1	0.38-0.48	0.58	4.3	77.1
ethyl ether	1.352							
ethyl formate	1.358							
ethyl propionate	1.382							
ethylene dichloride	1.445	230	0.79	9.7	0.38	0.49	3.7	83.5
formamide	1.450	210	3.3-3.76				7.3	210.5
heptane	1.385							
hexanone, 2-	1.395							
i-butyl acetate	1.388							
i-butyl alcohol			3				3.9	117.7
i-butyl formate	1.383							
i-butylamine	1.395							
i-octane	1.404	197-210	0.5	7	0.01	0.01	0.4	99.2
i-propyl acetate	1.375							
i-propyl ether	1.368	220	0.33-0.37	7.3	0.22	0.28	2.2	68.3

Appendix 1 contd...

Solvent	ri	UV cutoff	Viscosity (cP) at 20°C	Hildebrand solubility parameter	E° SiO$_2$	E° Al$_2$O$_3$	polarity index (Snyder)	BP (°C)
methanol	1.329	205	0.6	13.7	0.73	0.95	6.6	64.7
methoxyethanol, 2-	1.401	220	1.72			0.74	5.7	124.6
methyl acetate	1.362	260	0.37-0.45	9.2	0.46	0.6	4.4	56.3
methyl ethyl ketone (MEK)	1.379	330	0.43	9.3	0.39	0.51	4.5	80
methyl n-butyrate	1.391							
methyl-1-propanol, 2-	1.394							
methyl-2-butanone, 3-	1.386							
methyl-2-pentanone, 4-	1.394							
methyl-2-propanol, 2-	1.383							
methylene chloride	1.424	233	0.44	9.7	0.32	0.42	3.4	39.8
methylhexane, 2-	1.382							
methylhexane, 3-	1.386							
methylpentane, 2-	1.369							
methylpentane, 3-	1.374							
n-decane	1.412	210	0.92	7.8		0.04	0.3	174.1
n-hexane	1.375	195	0.313	7.3	0.03	0.01	0	68.9
Nitrobenzene			2.03				4.5	210.8
Nitroethane	1.392	380	0.68				5.3	114
Nitromethane	1.380							

Appendix 1 *contd...*

Solvent	ri	UV cutoff	Viscosity (cP) at 20°C	Hildebrand solubility parameter	E° SiO_2	E° Al_2O_3	polarity index (Snyder)	BP (°C)
nitropropane, 2-	1.392							
octafluoro-1-pentanol	1.316							
Octane	1.395		0.5				0.4	99.2
pentanone, 2-	1.390							
pentanone, 3-	1.390							
propanol, 1-			2.3				4.3	97.2
propanol, 2-	1.380	210+	2.35			0.82	4.3	82.4-117.7
Propionaldehyde	1.371							
propionic acid	1.386							
Propionitrile	1.366							
propyl ether	1.379							
propyl formate	1.375							
propylamine	1.386							
propyl acetate	1.382							
pyridine	1.510	305-330	0.94	10.7		0.71	5.3	115.3
t-butanol	1.385							
t-butyl methyl ether	1.370	210	0.27		0.35		2.9	55.2
Tetrahydrofuran	1.408	212-230	0.55	9.1	0.35	0.45	4.2	66

76

Appendix 1 *Contd...*

Solvent	ri	UV cutoff	Viscosity (cP) at 20°C	Hildebrand solubility parameter	E° SiO_2	E° Al_2O_3	polarity index (Snyder)	BP (°C)
Toluene	1.496	285	0.59	8.9	0.23	0.29	2.3	101.6
triethyl amine	1.401		0.38				1.8	89.5
trifluoroacetic acid	1.283							
Trifluoroethanol	1.290							
Trifluoropropanol	1.381							
trimethylbutane, 2,2,3-	1.387							
trimethylhexane, 2,2,5-	1.397							
trimethylpentane, 2,2,4-	1.389							
Valeronitrile	1.395							
Water	1.333	180	1	21		large	9	100
xylene, p-			0.7				2.4	138
Heptane	1.385	210						59

3   Preparative Chromatography

Introduction

Preparative chromatography is a very indistinct term as its meaning will be implied based upon the purpose of its use. For a botanist the term preparative chromatography may mean isolation of few grams of a phytoconstituents. For a forensic analyst it may mean the separation of only a few micrograms of substances for their characterization and to a biochemist, it may mean the segregation of a few milligrams of a substance essential for evaluating its pharmacological activity. Thus, the quantity of a substance that is separated does not establish whether the separation process can be termed as a preparative technique or not. Nevertheless, all preparative separations involve the *collection of an eluted substance* and does not only comprise of quantitative peak profile monitoring and measurement. It should be noted that the technique of chromatography, as invented by Tswett was not originally developed for quantitative purposes, but for the separation of specific pigments from extracts of plants. But, the earlier claims of chromatography were solely for preparative reasons until the development of gas chromatography (GC) that was used first used for analytical purposes.

Liquid column chromatography has originated from a preparative procedure and is now developed into an analytical technique, popularly known as high performance liquid chromatography (HPLC), which has led to the development of GC. In the earlier years, column loads were improved for preparative uses by expanding the dimensions of the column in GC and in HPLC. However, this approach has some limitations.

Preparative Thin Layer Chromatography (P-TLC)

In contrast to the analytical TLC, Preparative TLC is used to separate compounds of interest in a large amount ranging from a few milligrams to grams. Several planar chromatographic techniques are available to the botanical chemists. Some of these involve the movement of mobile phase through stationary phase by capillary action and some are forced flow methods such as centrifugal TLC and over pressure layer chromatography.

It is one of the efficient separation techniques that require the least of financial inputs and is carried out with the help of some basic equipment. Although the technique is still used in preliminary analysis in labs, it still has several drawbacks involved.

Basic Parameters in the Process of P-TLC

- *Adsorbents / Stationary Phase*

  Although many studies have been carried out to study the effect of thickness of adsorbent layer on the type of separation, the most frequently used thickness is 0.5-2 mm. The dimension of a preparative TLC plate is generally 20 × 20 mm or 20 × 40 mm. The limitation on the size of plate and thickness of sorbent (stationary phase) layer reduces the amount of material separated on PTLC. The maximum amount of sample that can be loaded on a TLC of 1.0 mm thickness is about $5mg/cm^2$. Silica gel is the most widely used adsorbent material for lipophilic and hydrophilic substances. For uniform and crack free layer preparation a number of sorbents are available commercially. The particle size and pore sizes of these commercially available sorbents are equivalent to TLC gradesorbents. The pre-coated plates for P-TLC can be purchased or prepared manually. The advantage of using handmade plates is that one can select any adsorbent material and desired thickness can be adopted. Spreaders manufactured by Camag and Degas are available commercially (Fig. 3.1).

- *Sample Application*

  One of the most critical aspects of a P-TLC process is the sorbent application. The plates to be used for coating should be prewashed in order to wash off and minimize the impurities. The impurities might adhere to the surface and when scrapped along with the compound of interest from the sorbent can cause possible interferences. For application on TLC plate the sample is dissolved in small amount of solvent. Generally, a volatile solvent (hexane, DCM or ethyl acetate) is preferred over less volatile solvents to avoid band broadening. The concentration of sample should be about 5-10%. During application utmost care is taken to apply the band as narrow as possible as it affects the resolution of components. For bands that are too broad, the concentration of band is brought about by migration of a polar solvent 2 mm above the band.   The plate is then dried and then the desired solvent system is allowed to run on the plate. Special pre-coated plates by 'Analtech' with concentration zones are also available commercially. These concentration zones are made up of an inert adsorbent strip material or a chemically bonded C_{18} layer. These are wedge shaped plates that enhance the resolution of sample zones.

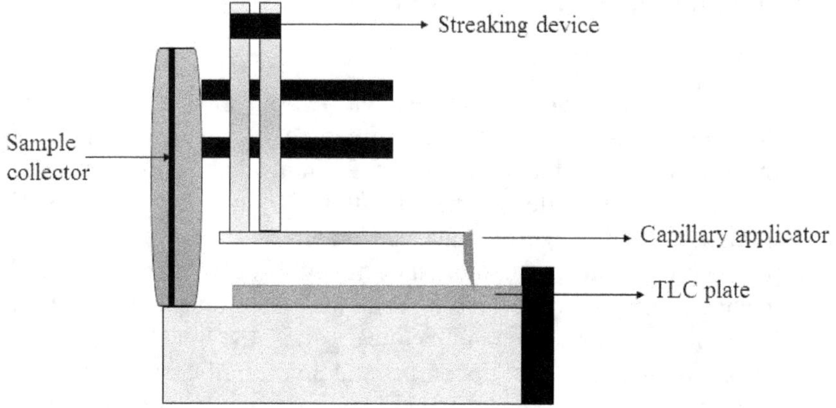

Figure 3.1 Spreader used for P-TLC plate

- ***Choice of Mobile Phase and Development of PTLC***

There are many variables in the process of development of a PTLC plate, but as generally 10-100 mg of a substance can be separated on a silica gel or aluminium oxide layer of 1mm thickness and 20 × 20 mm dimension. Doubling thickness of the sorbent layer allows 50% more of sample loading. Choice of solvent system is based by a preliminary investigation of analytical TLC. As the particle sizes are almost the same, a TLC profile is reproducible on P-TLC.

Hexane – ethyl acetate, hexane-acetone and chloroform-methanol are the most widely used binary mobile phases (in varying proportions) for PTLC separations. Addition of acetic acid or diethyl amine in small amounts helps in better resolution of acidic and basic compounds respectively.

Development of P-TLC plates is generally carried out in large glass tanks which can accommodate several plates for development at a time. The development tank is saturated with mobile phase and a filter paper dipped in the solvent. When a P-TLC is developed, a plate is dried and the R_f of the compound is estimated.

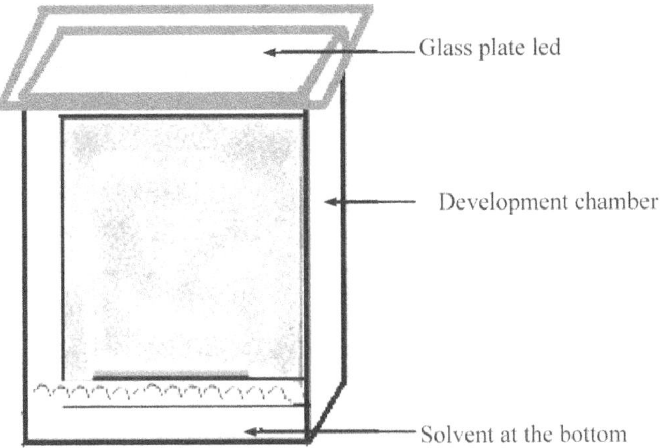

Figure 3.2 Development chamber of P-TLC plates

- ***Isolation of separated substance***

The band of interest is located with the help of known R_f value or by spotting a reference standard on the same plate in the same chromatographic run. The selected band is then separated with a spatula or tubular scrapper connected to vacuum collector. However, the use of vacuum for scrapping is not practicable for compounds that are sensitive as stream of air is in continuous contact with the purified product in the adsorbent material, and can cause auto oxidation. Irrespective of the collection method, the substance has to be extracted from sorbent by least polar solvent (about 5 ml solvent for 1 g substance). The longer duration of time that the substance is in contact with stationary phase, greater are the chances of decomposition of the substance. The extract is filtered through a glass frit of porosity 4 and then through a 0.25 mm- 0.45µm membrane.

Methanol is generally not used for extraction of separated substances as it can solublise silica gel and some of its impurities to some extent. Ethanol, chloroform or acetone are good alternative solvents for extraction than methanol.

Many P-TLC adsorbents have a fluorescent indicator which helps in localization of separated bands as long as separated bands absorb UV light. Some adsorbents have the problem of reacting with some acids like acetic acid. For non-UV absorbing compounds the bands can be located spraying the plate with water (e.g. for saponins) or covering the plate on one edge with glass plate and spraying one edge with particular derivatising reagent. The conventional spraying apparatus used for P-TLC and analytical TLC is depicted in Fig. 3.3.

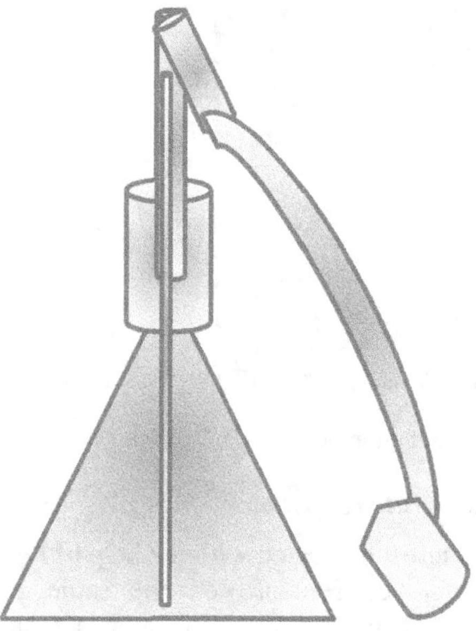

Figure 3.3 Diagrammatic representation of spraying bottle for P-TLC

- ***Impurities in Substance Separated by P-TLC***

  The compositions of binders and fluorescent indicators in P-TLC adsorbents are not generally known. These binders and indicators are extracted along with the compound of interest during the process. Higher the polarity of extracting solvent higher is the possibility of secondary material being extracted along with the desired compound. Another problem is that the binders and indicators used in sorbents do not absorb UV light and are generally missed in TLC profile of purified substance. Thus, a final purification step by Sephadex column is usually recommended to remove impurities like polyesters and phthalates.

Applications

- Screening of various extracts for e.g., antimicrobial and antioxidant activity or general toxicity. Fractions or compounds with significant activity can be detected directly on the TLC plate and subjected to further purification and/or identification steps.

- ***Impurity and Stability Testing of Synthetic Compounds:*** During synthesis of compounds, several intermediates, end products and impurities resulting due to addition of reaction solvents and modifiers can be identified and separated by employing preparative TLC. Stability of drugs exposed to various conditions of acid and base hydrolysis, photolysis, thermal degradation and oxidation can also be identified with preparative TLC.

- ***Separation Procedures of Organic, Inorganic, and Organometallic Compounds:*** Few examples where this technique has been employed in detection of organic, inorganic, and organometallic compounds are boron and thiocyanates from various soil and water samples, nitrites and cyanides generated in molasses, magnesium found in alloys and borate in bakery products.

- ***Identification of Vitamins, Foods and Beverages:*** The identification of fat-soluble vitamins, amino acids, carbohydrates, organic acids, and anthocyanins has been carried out in food products by use of preparative TLC. 2-hydroxycinnamaldehyde, a constituent of cinnamon, oleic acid phenacyl esters, *cis*-vaccenic and petroselinic acids found in oils of seeds, fatty acids found in commercially available spreads and triacylglycerols occurring in milk fat, have been reported to be analyzed by preparative TLC.

- ***Detection of Phytoconstituents in Plant Extracts:*** Various phytoconstituents like triterpenoids have been reported to be detected with preparative TLC. Plant species belonging to genus *Cassia* (*C. renigera*, *C. biflora* and *C. laevigata*) have been studied for their anti-fungal properties by detection of active constituents such as anthraquinone 1-carboxylic acid, by preparative TLC.

- ***Detection of Natural and Synthetic Food Colors:*** Natural organic and organic dyes and pigments extracted from extracts of the Indigo plant, rhizomes of ginger, logwood and teak plant, are reported to be identified and isolated by use of preparative TLC method. Mineral dyes identified by this technique also include yellow, brown and red from ocher, white dyes from limestone, black dyes from manganese, red colour dyes from cinnabar and lead oxide, green dyes from malachite and blue colour from azurite and lapis lazuli.

4   Thin Layer Chromatography (TLC)

Introduction

Chromatography is the process of separation of two or more compounds by distribution between two phases. One of the two phases is moving and the other is stationary. These two phases can comprise of solid-liquid, liquid-liquid or gas-liquid phases. Even if there are many different variations or techniques of chromatography, the principles are essentially the same. This chapter explores a very simple and basic technique for separating organic molecules - the thin-layer chromatography. Thin-layer chromatography or TLC is a form of chromatography where the stationary phase is normally a solid absorbent and the mobile phase can be a single solvent or combination of solvents.

Theory

In thin-layer chromatography, the stationary phase is a solid absorbent, usually finely ground alumina or silica gel that is coated (about 0.25 mm thick) on a supporting surface. The supporting surface can be made of glass slide (analytical scale) or plastic sheet. In many cases, a small amount of a binder such as plaster of Paris or Gypsum are mixed with the absorbent to facilitate the coating.

Thin layer chromatography is similar to paper chromatography techniques in which it involves spotting the mixture on the adsorbent layer and the solvent (mobile phase) is allowed to run upwards on the plate in a chromatographic tank/chamber. The advantage of TLC over paper chromatography in that its separations offer better resolution because of the much smaller size of the particles in the stationary phase.

The molecular level interaction of a TLC separation is illustrated in Fig. 4.1. The process involves a dynamic and rapid equilibrium of molecules between the two phases. As shown in Fig. 4.1, there are some "**free**" molecules of a component that are completely dissolved in the liquid or gaseous mobile phase and there are some "**adsorbed**" molecules of another component that stick on the surface of the solid stationary phase.

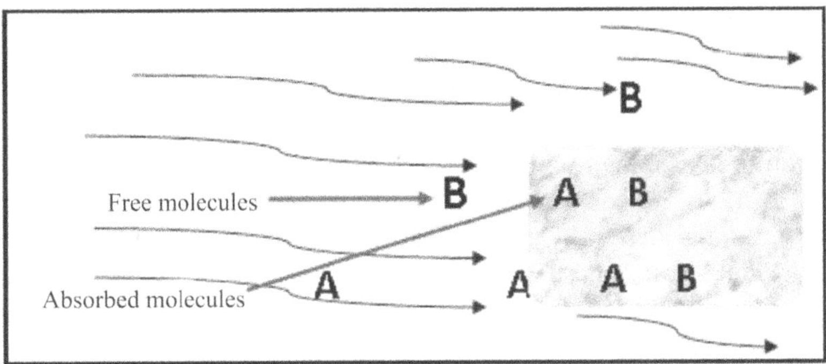

Figure 4.1 Mixture of A and B components of a mixture in mobile phase and absorbed on the stationary phase

Molecules continuously move back and forth between the free and absorbed states with numerous molecules absorbing and numerous other molecules desorbing at each time point. The equilibrium between the free and absorbed states depends on factors like polarity and size of the molecule, polarity of the stationary phase, polarity of the solvent.

Thus, an analyst has three different variables to modify in chromatography. The polarity of the molecules is determined by their functional groups. By selecting different stationary and mobile phases, one can alter the equilibrium between the free and absorbed states.

The equilibria between the solid and liquid phase is not the same as different molecules partition differently between the free and absorbed state. As shown in Fig. 4.2, molecule 'A' is weakly absorbed, its equilibrium lies in the direction of the free state and there is a higher concentration in the mobile phase. Whereas, molecule B, is strongly absorbed, and its equilibrium lies in the direction of the absorbed state, and it has a higher concentration on the stationary phase.

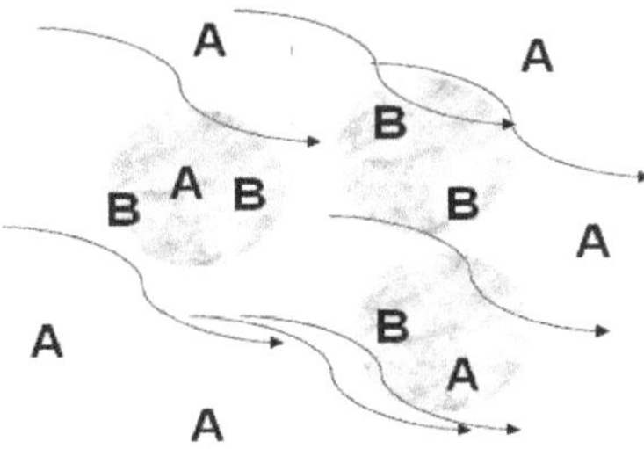

Figure 4.2 Dynamic equilibrium between the molecules A and B and the mobile and stationary phase

Only the addition of mixture to a combination of a mobile phase and a stationary phase does not separate it into its pure molecular components. For the process to happen, the mobile phase must flow past the stationary phase as depicted in Fig. 4.2. As the 'A' molecules spend more time in the mobile phase, they will be carried faster through the stationary phase and will move farther in a given period of time. However, since 'B' is absorbed to the stationary phase more than A, the B molecules spend less time in the mobile phase and hence move through the stationary phase particles comparatively more slowly.

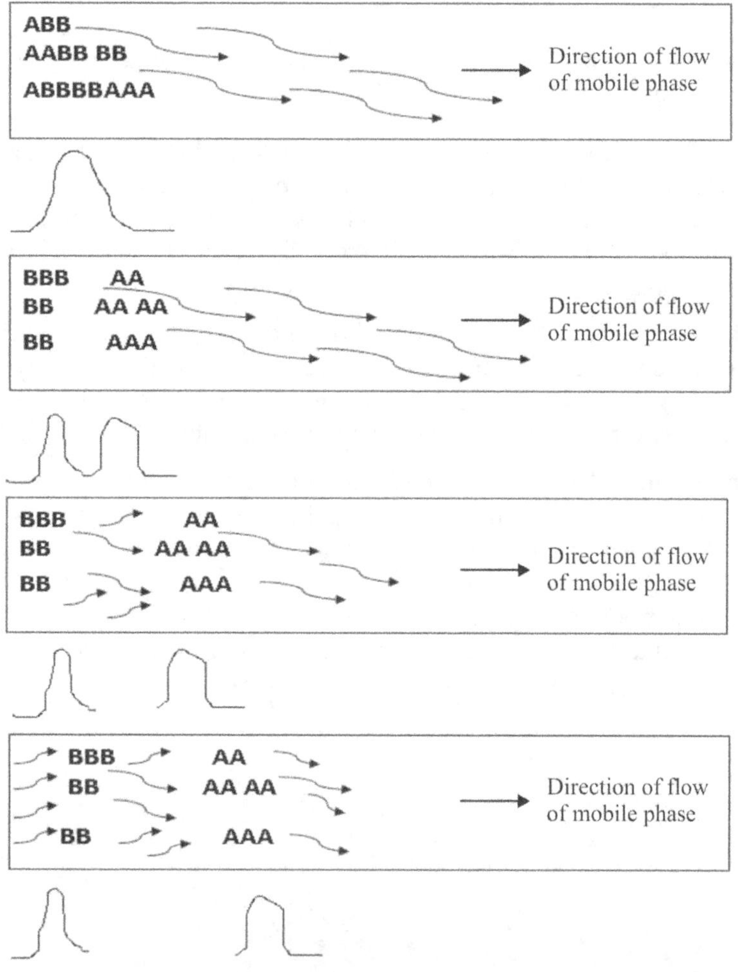

Figure 4.3 Mixture of A and B separated by a moving mobile phase while being absorbed on the stationary phase

The result of this flowing mobile phase is that A is steadily separated from B by moving further on in the flow. This separation process is depicted in Fig. 4.3.

The eluting solvent must also exhibit a maximum of selectivity in its ability to dissolve or desorb the substances being separated. When one substance is relatively soluble in a solvent, the result is that it can be eluted faster than another substance. Nevertheless, a more important property of the solvent is its ability to be itself adsorbed on the adsorbent. If the solvent is more strongly adsorbed than the components being separated, the solvent can take their place on the adsorbent and all the substances would flow together. And, if the solvent is less strongly adsorbed than the other components of the mixture, its involvement to different rates of elution will be only through its difference in solvent power towards them. And, if it is more strongly adsorbed than some components of the mixture and less strongly than others, the solvent system will greatly speed up the elution process of those substances that it can replace on the absorbent, without speeding up the elution of the others.

In TLC, the stationary phase is typically alumina $(Al_2O_3.xH2O)_n$ or silica gel $(SiO_2.xH_2O)_n$. The covalent networks of these absorbents construct very polar stationary phase materials.

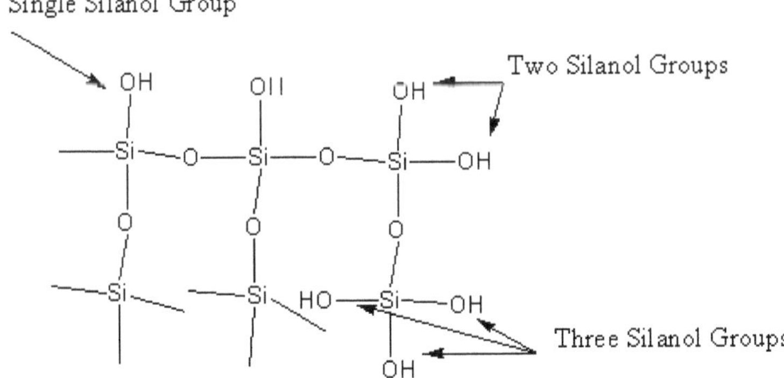

Figure 4.4 Structure of Silica gel

The electropositive character of the aluminum or silicon and the electronegative oxygen constitute a very polar stationary phase. Thus, the more polar the molecule to be separated, the stronger the attractive forces towards the stationary phase. The old proverb "like-dissolves-like" is applicable here. The polar stationary phase will more strongly attract polar molecules. Nonpolar molecules will have a lower attraction towards the stationary phase and they will remain in the solvent for a longer period of time. This is fundamentally how the phenomenon of partitioning separates the molecules. Separation is governed by the equilibrium but the component's affinity to the stationary phase versus the mobile phase determines the state of the equilibrium. Basically, the more polar the functional group, the stronger the bond to the stationary phase and slower is the movement of molecules. In most uncommon conditions, the molecules may not move at all. This difficulty can be overcome by increasing the polarity of the solvent system so that the equilibrium between the free and absorbed state is shifted towards the free. Although alumina and silica gel are the most widely stationary phases used for TLC, there are many other materials available stationary. These stationary phase materials range from paper to charcoal, nonpolar to polar, and reverse phase to normal phase.

Activated carbon (Charcoal, Nonit pellets)
Alumina (aluminum oxide, acidic, basic or neutral)
Magnesium oxide
Florisil (magnesium silicate)
Silica (silica gel)
Calcium sulfate Increasing Polarity
Starch
Cellulose   Increasing polarity
Paper
Reverse Phase (hydrocarbon-coated silica e.g. C-18)
Carbowax (polyethyleneglycol)
Cyanopropysiloxane
Methyl/Phenylsiloxane
Polydimethylsiloxane

Figure 4.5 List of common stationary phases with increasing polarity

As mentioned previously, the more polar compounds will adhere more strongly to the stationary phase as compared to the relatively less polar compounds. Several common compound classes according to how they will elute from silica or alumina are listed in Fig. 4.6.

Lowest/Slower (need polar mobile phase to elute

Sulfonic acids
Carboxylic acids
Phenols
Amines
Aldehydes
Ketones
Esters
Ethers
Aromatic halides Aromatic hydrocarbons
Dienes
Alkenes (Olefins)
Alkyl Halides (Halocarbons)
Alkane Hydrocarbons

Increasing Functional Group Polarity

Highest/Fastest (elute with nonpolar mobile phase)

Elution sequence by Functional Group
(using Silica or Alumina TLC or Column Chromatography)

Figure 4.6 Elution Order for some common functional groups with Ssilica or alumina as stationary phase

It is important to have knowledge of the elutropic series (given in chapter-basics of chromatography), the functional groups of the compounds to have a proper selection of mobile phase for a mixture. If the mobile phase is not previously optimized, one should start with a nonpolar solvent such as hexane and monitor the separation. If the components of the mixture do not separate discretely, a slightly more polar solvent such as ether or ethyl acetate should be added to the hexane. The differences in the separation to the previous plate should be observed. In a large amount of cases a combination of these two solvents is the best solution. However, if the spots still stay at the bottom of the plate, more of the polar solvents should be added. If the spot runs to the solvent front very rapidly, then a more nonpolar solvent can be added to the mobile phase. However, one should bear in mind that chromatography is not an exact science and optimization of parameters for a chromatographic method is based on trial and error method.

Technique of Thin-Layer Chromatography

Performing a TLC analysis consists of a number of steps: preparing of TLC plate; marking the TLC plate; spotting the TLC plate; developing the TLC plate; visualizing the substance spots, and measuring the R_f values.

Preparation of TLC plate: TLC plates are commercially available, with standard particle size ranges and different stationary phase adsorbents to improve reproducibility. They are prepared by mixing the adsorbent, with a small amount of inert binder like calcium sulfate (gypsum) and water. This mixture is spread as thick slurry on an inert carrier sheet, like glass, aluminum foil, or plastic. The resultant plate is dried and *activated* by heating in an oven for thirty minutes at 110 °C. The thickness of the adsorbent layer is typically around 0.1-0.25 mm. For laboratory scale analytical purposes one can prepare plates in a similar way taking care about the application to be uniform and around 0.5-2.0 mm in thickness.

Marking the TLC plate: To carry out a TLC separation, the sample is applied to the plate, as a small spot at the bottom edge of the plate. Since a TLC plate can simultaneously run multiple mixtures at one time, it is very important to properly label the plate. A pencil is always used to mark a TLC plate since the graphite carbon is inert. If organic ink is used to mark the plate, it will chromatograph like any other organic compound and give inaccurate results.

Activating the TLC plate: The TLC plate is placed in an oven at 50-60°C for 15-20 minutes to "activate" it. Activation involves driving off water molecules that bond to the polar sites on the plate. The process improves efficiency of separation.

Spotting of sample: To spot the plate, sealed glass capillaries can be used. Graduated capillaries are available commercially for this purpose. The application may be made with a micropipette prepared by heating and drawing out a melting point capillary. One may have to spot the plate a couple of times to ensure the material is present. If excess of sample is applied, a poor separation will result. Smearing, smudging and spots that overlap will result make it difficult for an analyst to identify the separated components. Sample amount should be used as low as possible, since this will reduce tailing and overlapping of spots; the lower limit is the ability to visualize the spots in the developed chromatogram. The starting position can be indicated by making a small mark near the edge of the plate. The spot on the thin layer plate must be applied about 1 cm above the base of the plate (Fig. 4.7).

Development of plate: After the solvent from the applied spot has evaporated the plate is immersed in a chamber previously saturated with the mobile phase. The applied spot is not dried and it is below the level of solvent the sample will be washed off when in contact with the mobile phase in the development tank. The plate has to be placed vertically in the development tank with the edge to which the spot was applied down.

The chamber used for development of the plate (Fig. 4.8) can be a simple beaker covered with a watch glass, or a cork-stoppered bottle. The mobile phase is poured into the container to a depth of a few millimeters. The spotted plate is then placed in the container, spotted end down; taking care that the solvent level is below the spots. The solvent then slowly rises in the adsorbent of the stationary phase by capillary action. To obtain reproducible results, the atmosphere in the development chamber must be saturated with the solvent. This can be accomplished by pouring the mobile phase around in the container before any plates have been added. The atmosphere in the chamber is then kept saturated by keeping the container closed all the time except for the brief moment during which a plate is added or removed. The solvents evaporate and the vapors saturate the chamber/tank. Saturation of development chambers helps in faster development of plate, because as soon as the plate is placed in the chamber the solvents settle upon the surface of the plate. This reduces the time and amount of solvent required for development of the plate.

The solvent which is at the bottom of the container, then runs up on the layer of adsorbent, passes over the spot, and continues to carry the components. This results in the separation of the materials in the spot. When the solvent front has practically reached the top of the plate (approx. 1cm less than the top edge), the thin layer plate is removed from the container (Fig. 4.9).

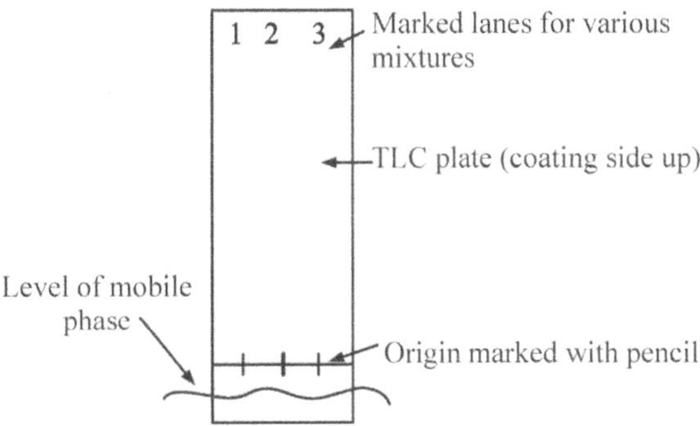

Figure 4.7 TLC plate for spotting

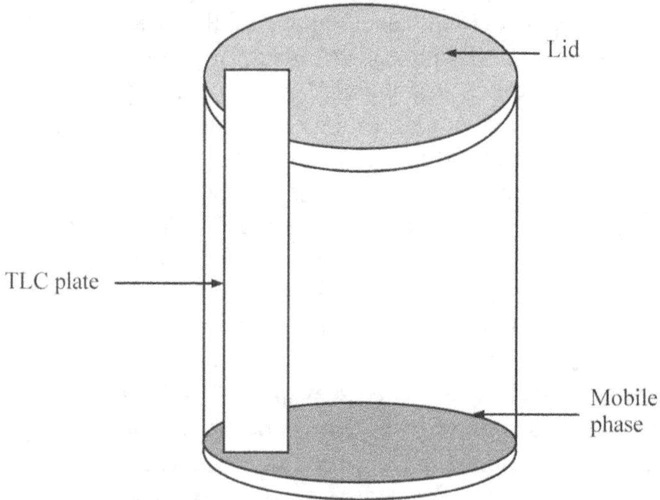

Figure 4.8 Development chamber for TLC plate

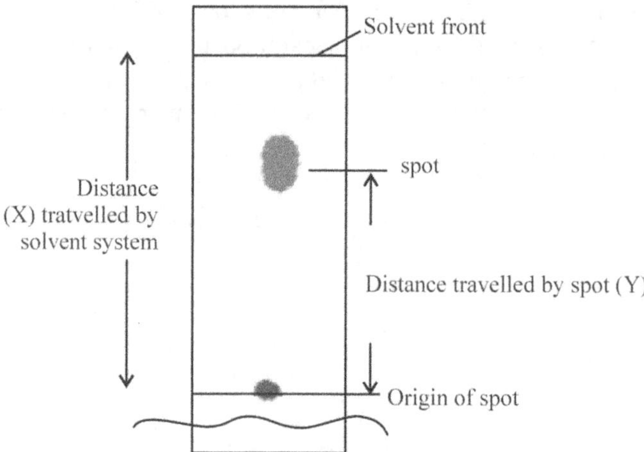

Figure 4.9 TLC Plate showing elution of a sample

As the amount of adsorbent involved is relatively low, and the ratio of adsorbent to sample must be high, the amount of sample must be very low (much less than a milligram). For this reason, thin-layer chromatography (TLC) is usually used as an analytical technique rather than a preparative.

Visualization: Once the development of the plate is completed (the solvent front has moved to within about 1 cm of the top end of the adsorbent), the plate should be removed from the developing chamber, the position of the solvent front should be marked, the solvent allowed to evaporate and the plate must be air dried. If the separated components of the applied sample are colored, they can be seen directly. Some organic compounds are colored and it is easy to visualize spots of organic compounds like dyes, inks or indicators. Nonetheless, since most organic compounds are colorless, direct visualization is not always possible. In most cases UV light is used in observing the separated spots. TLC plates contain an inorganic fluorescent indicator (usually manganese-activated zinc silicate) added to the silica gel which makes the TLC plate glow green under UV light of wavelength 254 nm. Compounds that can absorb UV light will quench the green fluorescence exhibiting a dark purple or bluish spots on the plate, which can be observed by keeping the plate under UV light and the compounds become visible to the naked eye (Fig. 4.10). The position of spots can be marked with pencil to have a record for further calculation of R_f values.

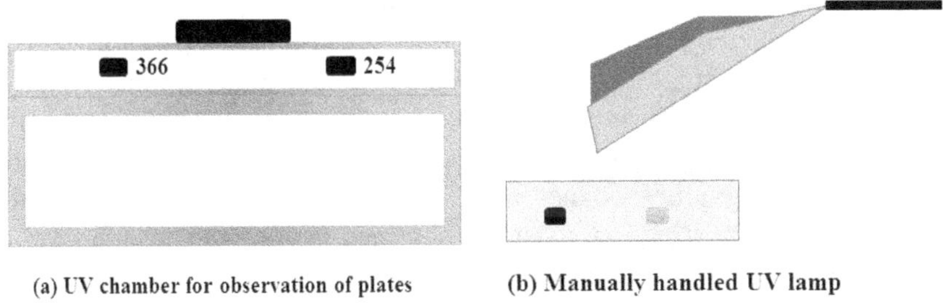

(a) UV chamber for observation of plates   (b) Manually handled UV lamp

Figure 4.10 Visualization of spots using UV light

Another technique for visualization is using an iodine (I2) chamber. However, Iodine is a nonspecific reagent for detection. Specific reagents are available for various compounds, depending upon the chemical nature of the sample under investigation, for example 0.2% ninhydrinin ethanol for visualizing amino acid spots. Apart from Iodine other reagents used for detection are Potassium permanganate – oxidation, and Bromine.

Iodine on sublimation and in the vapour phase gets adsorbed to organic molecules on the plate. The organic spots on the plate turn brown in color and can be easily visualized. These observed spots can be marked with a pencil as over a period of time, the adsorbed iodine will evaporate and the location of spots would not be possible. Some compounds that do not absorb UV light at the wavelength of 254 nm times, need to be observed with Iodine. Using both methods (UV light and Iodine) will ensure correct identification of all the spots on the TLC plate.

Calculation of R_f values: In addition to qualitative data, TLC can also provide a chromatographic measurement known as an R_f value. The R_f value is the "retardation factor" or the "ratio-to-front" value expressed as a decimal fraction.

The R_f value can be calculated as (shown in Fig. 4.9):

$$R_f \text{ value} = \frac{\text{Distance travelled by solute /spot (y)}}{\text{Distance travelled by solvent system/mobile phase (x)}}$$

This value can be calculated for every component spot observed on a TLC plate. It basically describes the distance traveled by the individual components. If two spots travel the same distance or have the same R_f value then one may conclude that the two components are the same molecule. For such investigations of R_f value comparisons to be valid; the TLC plates must be run under the same chromatographic conditions. The parameters of chromatographic conditions include the stationary phase, mobile phase, and temperature. It is likely that many organic compounds have the same melting point and color, and can have the same R_f value, thus identical R_f values do not necessarily mean identical compounds. Supplementary information must be obtained before one can arrive to such a conclusion. It is essential to restate that R_f values are only significant when the same chromatographic conditions are used.

Problems in TLC

Over-large Spots: Sample spots made using TLC capillaries should not be larger than 1-2 mm in diameter in size, as the component spots in the developed plate will be usually larger than, the size of the initial spot. Thus, components may not be well resolved and the spots may overlap considerably and may appear to be one large spot. Small initial spots, lead to well separated components.

Uneven Advance of Solvent Front: The solvent front may appear to bow either up or down in the center, instead of a straight linear appearance. Uneven movement of mobile phase leads to uneven movement of spots of the substance, resulting to inaccurate R_f values.

A common cause of irregular solvent move on is the use of a developing chamber that does not have a flat bottom. If the bottom of the TLC plate is placed on this curved surface, the shape of the solvent advance line will be affected. It is therefore important to use flat-bottomed developing chambers in TLC. A curved solvent front may also result if very little developing solvent is placed in the chamber; if the plate is not cut properly, and if the plate is excessively tilted in the chamber. Thus, extreme care should be taken in choosing a chamber for development to avoid curved solvent fronts. Water is rarely used as a solvent in mobile phase for TLC because it has a tendency to produce a significantly curved front, which may be due to its unusually high surface tension.

Streaking: Sometimes a spot may move along a TLC plate as a long streak, rather than as a single discrete spot. This may result due to spotting of the plate with excess of substance, more than the mobile phase can handle. The mobile phase carries as much substance as it can, but a considerable amount of substance is left behind. Then this excess of substance will be dragged along by the solvent leaving a trail. Streaking can be reduced by diluting the spotting solution until development and visualization show satisfactory results instead of streaks.

Applications of TLC

TLC is a quick and economical microscale technique that can be used for a variety of applications like:

- *Determination of the number of components in a mixture:* TLC can be used for analysis of numerous phytoconstituents present within a particular plant extract or a complex mixture of food based products, herbal formulations or dyes etc.

- *Identification of a substance:* Substances can be analyzed with TLC method by employing pre and post chromatographic derivatising techniques or by comparison with reference standards. Compounds like sterols, phenols, flavonoids and terpenes are identified by derivatization.

- *To check progress of organic reactions:* The reaction process in synthesis of organic products is monitored by TLC analysis of the starting material, the reaction intermediates and the end products. Examples include, conversion of esters to aldehydes, 2,2'-bis (diphenylphosphino)-1,1'-binaphthyl synthesis from 2-napthol.

- *To determine appropriate conditions for column chromatography:* The sequence of elution of components from column chromatography, their type and identity can be checked by using TLC for the eluents/ fractions collected.

- *In forensic work, for example in the separation of dyes from fibres:* Acidic, direct and metallized dyes from fibres like wool, silk, polypropylene, and polyamides are extracted by pyridine/water andcan be analyzed by TLC method. Azoic dyes are extracted with pyridine/water from cotton, viscose and modified acrylic fibers.

Explained below is anexample of TLC analysis of Amino Acids: TLC analysis of amino acids is more difficult than TLC of inks, as amino acids are colorless. Thus, one cannot monitor their progressive movement up the plate, and cannot see the spots with the naked eye after the plate is fully developed. To detect the spots, it is necessary to use either the ninhydrin (specific reagent for amino acids) or the black-light visualization techniques (UV lamp). The latter can be used only if one uses fluorescent TLC plates. Until the spots are visualized one will not be able to estimate whether or not a chosen solvent system has been effective in moving an amino acid. The process of optimizing an effective solvent system requires the knowledge of basics of chromatography.

As a point of general information, amino acids are quite polar and they will be inclined to move on silica gel plates with polar solvents. They have R_f values close to 1 when water or concentrated ammonia is used as the mobile phase, possibly because of their high solubility in water. Addition of a less polar solvent a with polar will yield smaller R_f values, roughly in proportion to the amount of less polar solvent used. Alanine, glycine, threonine, and proline all have R_f values of approximately 0.60 when developed with a 50/50 mixture of water and n-propanol, and around 0.40 when developed with a 30/70 mixture of concentrated NH_3 and n-propanol. The below mentioned procedure presumes the use of 50/50 water/n-propanol as the mobile phase, but one can always have a trial with other polar/non-polar combinations of solvents.

Experimental Procedure: In the hood, 10 mL of mixture consisting of 50% 1-propanol and 50% water by volume is prepared. About half of this is poured into a clean developing tank. In a 1-dram vial, a solution of about 0.001 g of the selected amino acid in 0.2 ml of water is prepared.

The amino acid is dissolved in it and, some solution is then drawnup in a spotting capillary. The spots are applied on a properly marked and activated TLC plate. The plate is allowed to dry for 5 minutes, and then carefully placed into the developing tank so that its bottom is submerged in the developing solvent. The lid is closed and the plate is allowed to develop until solvent has risen to the marked line at the top of the plate. The plate is removed from the tank and placed in an oven at $50^{\circ}C$ to dry. When the plate is dry, the spots are visualized using ninhydrin spray or iodination. The amino acid spots are marked with pencil, and R_f values are calculated. The measured R_f values are compared with the values posted for the amino acids.

On this basis, one can constrict the process of identification of a particular amino acid. In combination with other data that is available with this information one can unambiguously identify an amino acid. Suppose that the selected amino acid has an R_f value similar to that of, standard alanine. One should then prepare a small amount of standard alanine solution and spot it alongside with the sample (test) amino acid on a new single TLC plate. If, the test amino acid has exactly the same R_f value as standard alanine, and it has the same shape and color it confirms that both the amino acids are the same.

Concluding, it is very important to be observant of every detail in doing TLC. In addition to the R_f values, the shapes of the spots produced by a particular developing solvent and the shade of color produced by iodine or ninhydrin can be distinctive for that substance. When alanine, glycine, threonine, and proline are applied side-by-side on a TLC plate and developed with 70% n-propanol/30% conc. NH_3, the following observations can be made:

Table 4.1 TLC characteristics of amino acids with different developing solvents

Amino Acid	Solvent	Spot Color after Iodination	Spot Color with Ninhydrin	R_f Value	Spot Shape
alanine	30/70 conc. NH_3/n-propanol	white on brown background	purple	0.38	elongated oval
alanine	50/50 water/n-propanol	white on brown background	purple	0.65	Circle
glycine	30/70 conc NH_3/n-propanol	white on brown background	pink	0.25	elongated oval
glycine	50/50 water/n-propanol	white on brown background	pink	0.55	Circle

Table 4.1 *Contd...*

Amino Acid	Solvent	Spot Color after Iodination	Spot Color with Ninhydrin	R_f Value	Spot Shape
threonine	30/70 conc. NH₃/n-propanol	white on brown background	purple	0.41	elongated oval
threonine	50/50 water/n-propanol	white on brown background	purple	0.57	Circle
proline	30/70 conc. NH₃/n-propanol	dark brown on brown background	yellow with pink border	0.39	elongated oval
proline	50/50 water/n-propanol	white on brown background	yellow with pink border	0.65	Circle

The polarity basics discussed in this chapter can be useful in many different types of chromatography including: Column Chromatography, Gas Chromatography, and High Performance Liquid Chromatography (HPLC). The details will be dealt in the following chapter.

5

High Performance Thin Layer Chromatography (HPTLC) and Hyphenated Techniques

Introduction

High Performance Thin layer Chromatography (HPTLC) is an advanced progression of TLC. It is also referred to as Modern Thin-Layer Chromatography, High Pressure chromatography or Instrumental Thin-Layer Chromatography. It renders a number of advantages over the conventional TLC process due to its attributes of speed of analysis, low cost of analysis, high throughout analysis, and complete automation. Other advantages include the feasibility of post and pre-chromatographic derivatisation, availability of various types of stationary phase that are disposable, feasibility of repetition of densitometric evaluation, storage of densitometry analysis data, image capturing of fingerprints, considerable level of analyte sensitivity in detection and quantitation of analytes post detection.

This technique offers better separation and resolution due to the precoated commercially available plates that have layers with optimized uniform absorbent surface and smaller particle size. Pressure is applied during sample application and drying and it thus decreases the total time for analysis and development. Furthermore the process can be automated depending upon the user's needs for autosampling, and mixing of solvents for mobile phases. The built in detection system for chromatograms and software for computing the stored data adds to the advantages of the technique. These are the reasons why HPTLC has a significant importance in Planar chromatography analysis and is used as a versatile technique.

HPTLC Steps and Procedures

The various steps involved in an HPTLC analysis are sample application, development of plates, derivatisation (if essential) and densitometric evaluation. Each of the steps are described below in brief.

Prewashing of Plates/Stationary Phases

The stationary phase materials on the HPTLC plates are prone to moisture and impurities in the atmosphere. Thus the plates should be stored in dehumidified chambers and care should be taken while handling that the application surfaces should not be touched with hands to avoid transfer of impurities. The plates should be held only at the edges to prevent contamination. To remove any possible impurities the plates should be pre-washed overnight with methanol, by allowing the methanol to run over the plates in a twin trough chamber so that the impurities are eluted towards the edge. The plates can then be dried in an oven at 120^0C for 20 min or lesser. Care should be taken not to overheat the plates as heating would distort the plate dimensions if they are aluminium backed.

Application of Samples

The samples are applied as bands on pre-coated or prepared plates with the help of semiautomatic or fully automatic application devices. Commercially available applicators from *CAMAG* are *Linomat 5, Automatic TLC sampler* III and IV. The sample volumes and band widths can be selected based upon the needs of the analysis. During application, a spray of nitrogen through the application port helps in conditioning of the band by instant drying of the solvent and avoiding broadening of bands. A typical HPTLC applicator is shown in Fig. 5.1. Graduated Hamilton syringes are used for the application of samples on precoated plates where the quantities as low as microlitres can be adjusted. For higher sample load or for specific analysis when samples are to be applied as spots, pipettes with 100 nL and 200 nL capacities and fixed volumes are available. These *Nanopipettes*serve a good aspect when a particular volume of sample is to be dispensed, however accuracy is not as good as the Hamilton syringes. *Glass capillaries* can be used for larger volumes of sample application. These capillaries have a good volume precision and are transparent and disposable.

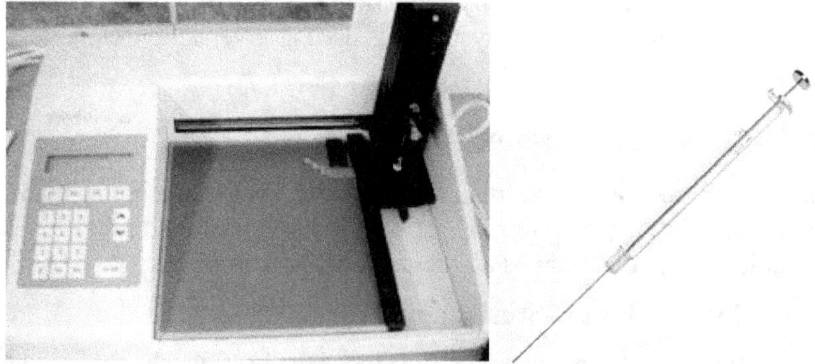

Figure 5.1 A HPTLC applicator device and Hamilton syringe

Development of HPTLC Plates

The conventional method of developing a plate is by immersing the bottom edge of a HPTLC plate in a development chamber that is pre-saturated with mobile phase. The mobile phase travels on the plate by capillary action. As mentioned in earlier chapters the pre-saturation of development chamber with mobile phase helps in faster and effective development of the plate. Pre-saturation is helpful where polar solvents like water, methanol, and acids or bases are used. Some analysts line a filter paper soaked with solvent system for saturation process. If a counter-plate is placed instead opposite to the developing plate in a twin trough chamber, it is called *"sandwich-configuration"*.

A *twin trough* chamber is more appropriately used for development of HPTLC plates where the base is slightly elevated and is divided into two parts. Such a chamber helps in simultaneous development of two plates (if mobile phases are identical) and favors less mobile phase consumption due to the raised wedge shaped bottom. *Horizontal chamber* development is also carried out in HPTLC process where the sample bands are applied parallel to both opposing sides of the plates, and the plate is developed from the opposite edges headed for the centre. This method helps in analysis of double number of samples. Nowadays, Automatic developing chambers (ADC) are also available and these have complete automation for control of plate drying, mobile phase run (development), preconditioning, etc. with the help of a computer based programmed unit.

Derivatization

The step of derivatisation can be carried out for substances that are not visible to naked eye or UV light at long-wave UV light 366 nm and short-wave UV light 254 nm. This step converts the non-detectable compounds into detectable or visible ones and improves detectability or induces fluorescence. Various sprayers are available for spraying the derivatising reagent on the plate. The selection of particular compound or constituent will depend upon the chemistry of the analyte. Commonly used derivatising agents are sulphuric acid, ferric chloride solution, vanillin sulphuric acid reagent. The derivatising agent can be sprayed or the plate can be dipped into the solution for few seconds for derivatising. The dipping / immersion method is preferred over spraying method to ensure uniformity of the spread of the reagent and hence a proper quantitative evaluation can be performed. Some reagents require heating of the plate for proper detection after dipping of the plate into the solution.

UV Cabinet for Visualization

The UV cabinet is an essential part of the instrumentation required for HPTLC analysis. It is equipped for visualization at 366 nm, 254 nm and in white light. At 366 nm the substances that can be excited to fluoresce can be seen. The spots appear as bright different colored bands against a dark background. When viewed under 254 nm substances that absorb UV light become visible, if the stationary phase material of the plate contains a fluorescent indicator. Various stationary phase materials like silica gel, keiselguhr, alumina etc. are available with or without binders and fluorescent indicators. The binders are usually made up of gypsum or poly (vinyl pyrrolidone) and fluorescent indicators are made from manganese-activated zinc silicate may that help in visualization of analytes by fluorescence quenching. A picture of UV cabinet for visualization of HPTLC plate is shown in Fig. 5.2.

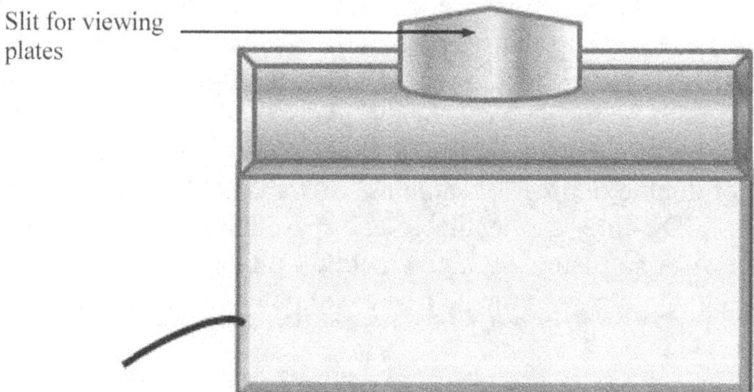

Figure 5.2 UV cabinet for visualization of HPTLC plates

Chromatogram Evaluation

After development of plates, the chromatograms of analytes can be evaluated either under ultraviolet or white light. One may choose for visual inspection, processing of images after recording, performing video densitometric analysis and documentation for quantitative estimation with monochromatic light in a densitometer. The bands of the plate are placed in scanner and the densitometric evaluation (indicated in Fig. 5.3) occurs with the help of optics, detectors and other accessories. The raw data obtained is used for integration of peaks and for generation of statistical data. The software's provided have a library of spectrum stored which can be used for comparison of spectra's of unknown compounds. Multiple wavelength scanning is also an added advantage of the software's used in HPTLC which helps scanning of chromatograms over a wide range of wavelengths. A typical HPTLC chromatogram is shown in Fig. 5.4, and Fig. 5.5 indicates the peak purity spectra obtained after densitometric Scanning. A picture of HPTLC Scanner is shown in Fig. 5.6.

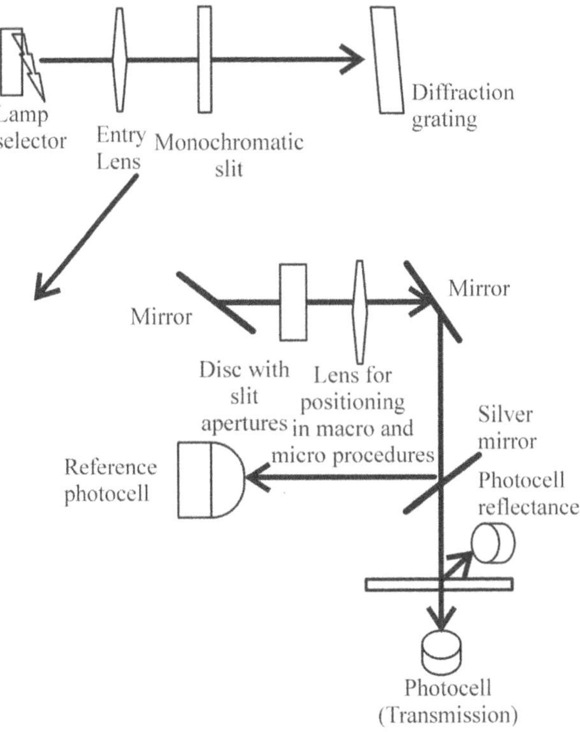

Figure 5.3 Schematic representation of instrumentation of densitometric scanning

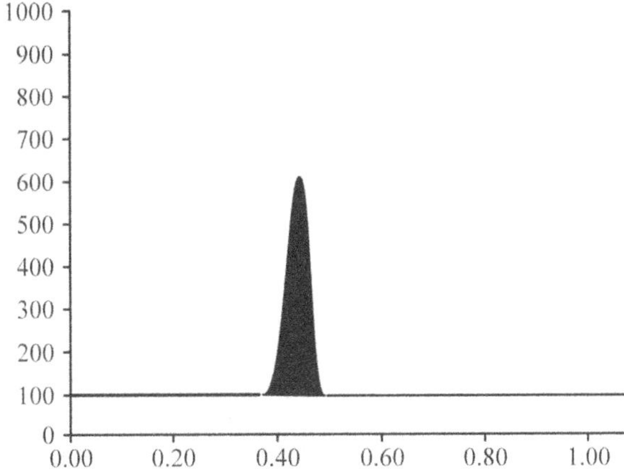

Figure 5.4 A typical HPTLC chromatogram

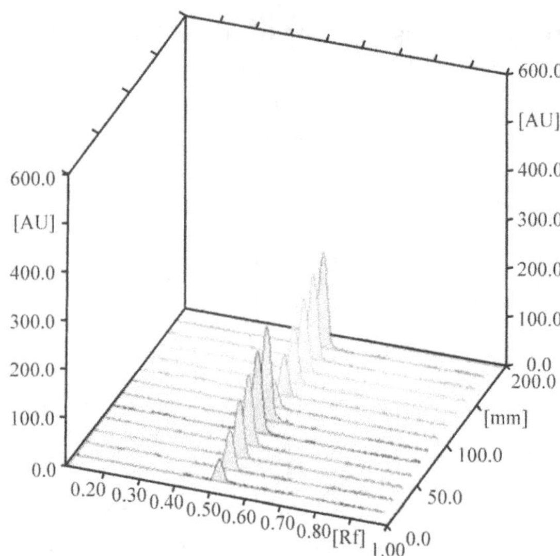

Figure 5.5 Peak purity spectra obtained after HPTLC Densitometric Scanning

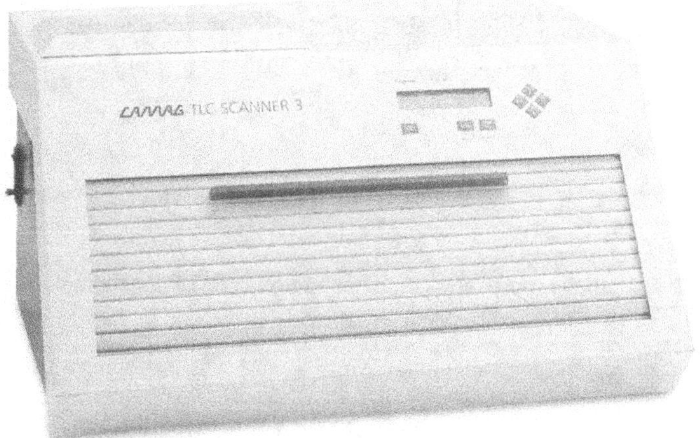

Figure 5.6 HPTLC Scanner

Applications of HPTLC

- *In the analysis of pharmaceutical formulations:* HPTLC has been used extensively in quality control of pharmaceutical dosage forms including tablets, capsules and syrups, to check the content uniformity, purity, identity and stability. Few examples of drugs analyzed by HPTLC include ethamsylate, mefenamic acid, mexiletine hydrochloride, olanzapine and etoricoxib.

- *In analysis of natural and organic synthetic products:* Like TLC, HPTLC has also been utilized for analyses of plant extracts, plant based formulations, reaction intermediates and end products in organic synthesis. It has also been used in stability testing, identification, and investigation of adulteration in herbal drug formulations.

- *For analysis food and food supplements:* HPTLC analysis has been used in analysis of food products to test additives (ex. vitamins), check stability and degradation products, shelf life and contamination.

- *In environmental studies:* HPTLC has been used to check the components in water, soil, industrial waste, and pesticides.

- *In analysis of cosmetics:* The presence of specific dyes, their concentrations and degradation products can be checked by HPTLC analysis. It is also used as an important technique to identify adulterants, raw material quality and preservatives in cosmetic formulations.

- *In analysis of clinical samples:* HPTLC can be employed in analysis of biological samples to identify metabolites, lipids in tissue samples, screening of drugs and control of doping.

Hyphenation in HPTLC

Since about a decade the hyphenation techniques have gained a tremendous importance in the analysis sector of pharmaceutical industries due to their ability of high throughput screening over a varied range of compounds. Planar chromatography has been hyphenated with high-performance Mass Spectroscopy (MS), Raman Spectroscopy (RS), High Performance Liquid Chromatography (HPLC), and Fourier transform infra-red (FTIR). The HPTLC instrument itself has the UV/visible diode array technique for determination of peak purity of analytes.

- **High Performance Thin Layer Chromatography-Mass Spectrometry (HPTLC–MS):** The coupling of chromatographic techniques with mass spectrometric detection is considered as a very useful innovation for analytical chemistry and finds its applicability in many fields of research. Mass spectrometric analysis gives additional data to aid the information about the identification of the compound obtained from chromatographic analysis. HPTLC-MS is used in limited manner by researchers as compared to LC-MS. A complete automation and interfacing of these two instrumentation techniques is a big challenge. However researchers at small scale level have tried to develop the interface by eluting the desired from the HPTLC plate and transferring it online into the mass spectrometer. In cases where the target zone is not visible it is marked under 254 nm or 366 nm wavelength and extrapolated for area after derivatisation of adjacent bands. The HPTLC-MS coupling operates in a semiautomatic manner and the data acquisition is carried out by flow injection analysis, a direct flow infusion or a placebo injection. This is then followed by a cleaning step and later the setup can be used for next analysis. The hyphenation of HPTLC and MS holds a great promise in future research applications. It has been applied to analysis of amino acids, unknown impurities, and herbal drug analysis.

- **High Performance Thin Layer Chromatography-Infrared Spectroscopy (HPTLC-IR):** Infrared (IR) is used for the elucidation of molecular structures and estimation of characteristic absorption bands and can be used to distinguish closely related substances. The coupling of HPTLC and FTIR can be classified into two groups-indirect and direct type. In the Indirect coupling method the substance is transferred from a TLC band to a IR non absorbing material like KBr or KCl or the HPTLC bands are cut from the plate for in-situ measurement when the recording of spectra is carried out. The direct type of analysis was introduced by Glauninger in 1989. Prior to the introduction of this direct type the coupling of HPTLC and UV-VIS was the only available technique. However, the data obtained from UV-VIS spectra is relatively insufficient for identification of a substance. HPTLC-FTIR offers the advantage of quantification and detection of non-UV and UV absorbing substances and hence finds its place in a wide range of applications. This hyphenation is superior to other available hyphenated techniques and is used in forensic analysis, drug and food testing and environmental and biological testing.

TLC/MALDI Coupling

Coupled TLC/MALDI systems are commercially available and find their applicability in planar chromatography for numerous analyses. MALDI MS is known to be an "imaging" technique for fine slices of tissues where the test compound is dispersed in a "matrix" of other compounds and silica gel of HPTLC plate and then scanned. TLC/MALDI MS has several merits like: the data obtained from mass spectrum is more informative than R_f value, the information about spatial resolution can begained by MALDI MS. Irrespective of the sample size, the MALDI MS method requires that a UV-absorbing matrix is coated on the HPTLC plate and that the UV laser does not pass through into the plate, the compound must be removed from the base of the plate to the surface of the plate. There are various ways of applying MALDI matrix solution to the HPTLC plate: by adding drops of matrix solution on the desired spot, reducing spot size by use of solvents with high surface tension, spraying of matrix solution or pressing the crystallized matrix solution on TLC plate surface. Analysts prefer use of hybrid or special plates for analysis or fixing up the plate with adhesive onto a reference MALDI and loading it for mass spectrometric analysis. Aluminium backed plates are preferred for this type of analysis as the plate should allow electrical conductivity to permit desorption of ions from the plate, which may not be possible if glass backed plates are used.

6   HPLC and Related Hyphenated Techniques

Introduction

The technique of liquid chromatography was first discovered in the twentieth century and was initially used to separate colored compounds, after Mikhail Tswett coined the term *chromatography*. High Performance Liquid Chromatography (HPLC) is a type of chromatographic technique that utilizes a liquid mobile phase to separate the components of a mixture. The stationary phase is packed into a column and the components to be separated are dissolved in a suitable solvent and then forced to flow through a chromatographic column under a high pressure. The separation of components occur in the column. The resolution of peaks of separated components is dependent upon the degree of interaction between the solute components and the stationary phase. The interaction of the solute with mobile and stationary phases can be influenced by a number of factors and through different choices of both solvents and stationary phases. Thus, HPLC finds a well accepted place amongst other chromatographic techniques as it has a high degree of versatility, that is not found in other chromatographic techniques and it has the ability to easily separate complex sample mixtures.

HPLC Theory

HPLC technique is an active adsorption process. When the analyte molecules move through the porous column bed, the analyte molecules have a tendency to interact with the surface adsorption sites. There may be different types of the adsorption forces included in the process of retention, based upon the mode of HPLC used for analysis.

Hydrophobic (non-specific) interactions are the forces active in **reversed-phase (RP) type of** separations. In the **normal phase (NP)** separations the dipole-dipole (polar) interactions are predominant. The ionic interactions are accountable for the retention process occurring in **ion-exchange** chromatography.

In all the types of above mentioned processes the interactions are competitive. However, in case of **SEC (size-exclusion chromatography),** the separation of analytes in a mixture depends upon the molecular size of its components. The larger the size of the molecule, the lesser is the possibility of the molecule to penetrate into the adsorbent pore space and will be retained longer. The attributes that make HPLC better as compared with the classical LC technique are the high resolution, column packing with small (3, 5 and 10 µm) particle sizes that increase the resolution; relatively higher inlet pressures and controlled flow of the solvent system; continuous flow detectors; high sensitivity and rapid analysis. "High pressure liquid chromatography" or HPLC is misunderstood to be called so due to use of high pressure in the process. However, in complete sense it is not true. The high performance is due to other factors like, sensitive detectors, fine particle size of stationary phase in column, accurate low volume injectors etc.

The general basics of liquid chromatography are elaborated in the previous chapters.

Instrumentation

HPLC instrumentation is very expensive due to the low tolerances and sensitivity of the separation process. In order to obtain reproducible results, the conditions of analysis must also be reproducible. Thus, the solvents and the accessories for HPLC must be of high quality.

HPLC instrumentation system comprises of a pump, injector, column, detector and data system. The most critical part of the system is the column where the separation takes place. In order to move the mobile phase through the micron sized pores in the column packing a high pressure pump is required. The process of separation is initiated by injecting the solution containing solute/analytes into the column. The mobile phase is pumped through the column and results in separation of components. The component eluted in the form of narrow bands from the column are detected by a suitable detector and the response of the detector to each component is displayed on the computer screen in the form of a chromatogram. A diagrammatic representation of HPLC unit is shown in Fig. 6.1.

- *Solvent System*

  The solvent system, or solvents, used in HPLC analysis are mixtures of polar and non-polar solvents with varying concentrations based about the type of the nature of analytes to be analysed. If the solvents used in HPLC are not of considerable purity they tend to block/plug the narrow bore of columns, thus, they must be free of dissolved gases or any particulate matter which may interfere during separation. Apart from the composition of the eluent that affects separation process other factors like purity, detector compatibility, solubility of the sample, viscosity, and chemical inertness affect separation. For reversed-phase separations the mobile phase is usually a mixture of water with some polar organic solvent such as acetonitrile or methanol and the normal phase mode, solvents are mainly nonpolar. In case of size-exclusion HPLC the mobile phase has to dissolve polymers, such that any possible interactions of the sample molecule and the surface of the packing material are avoided.

The use of buffers is also employed in certain separation in HPLC and LC-MS methods. Buffers are used when the analytes are ionizable, as ionization of analytes may cause a drastic change in the pH. If the pH of an acid is found 2 units above the *pKa*, it can lead to higher ionization and a pH of 2 units below the *pKa*, can cause analyte to remain unionized. Thus, buffers help maintain the pH of the solvent system and control the ionization of the analytes. The most suitable buffer system should be within ±1 unit of the *pKa*. Phosphate buffers are most widely used for HPLC analysis. However, other buffers like acetate, borate, citrate, ammonium bicarbonate and ammonium formate including several others can be used. Phosphate buffers can be used for UV detection below 220 nm wavelength and are thus most commonly used in HPLC separations. The phosphate buffer has 3 pH ranges: pH 1.1-3.1 (for *pKa* 2.1), pH 6.2 – 8.2 (for *pKa* 7.2) and pH 11.3 – 13.3 (for *pKa* 12.3). Practical considerations lead to elimination of the higher range and reduction of the lower pH range to 2.0 <pH<3.1. Thus, there arises a need for a buffer to compensate for the range between 3.8<pH<5.8. An acetate buffer provides the characteristic to fill up this range of pH that is not covered by phosphate buffers. Analysts prepare a mixture called as "Universal Buffer" by mixing 20 mm acetate and 20 mm phosphate buffer. The pH of the resultant mixture is then adjusted to the desired pH value in 2.0 ≤ pH ≤8.0 range. This strategy helps one to have a buffer that can be used for an entire pH range, ranging from 5.8 < pH < 6.2 down upto 3.1 < pH < 3.8.

- ***Stationary Phase***

HPLC separations depend much upon the surface interactions, and are affected by the types of the adsorption sites. Modern HPLC adsorbents are made up of small rigid porous particles with greater surface area. The suitable adsorbent parameters expected in a HPLC separation are its particle size (ranging from 3 to 10 μm), particle size distribution (as narrow as possible) and the chemical properties of the adsorbent surface. Based upon the type of the ligand attached to the surface, the adsorbent may be normal phase (-NH$_2$, -OH), or reversed-phase (C$_{18}$, C$_5$, C$_8$, CN, NH2), and anion (CH$_2$NR$_3{}^+$OH$^-$), or cation (R-SO$_3{}^-$H$^+$) exchangers.

If the interaction of a species is stronger with the adsorbent surface, it will spend more time in a column and will thus have a larger retention time. When columns are packed with solids such as silica or alumina; the columns are termed as *homogeneous columns*. If stationary phase in a column is made up of a liquid bonded to a solid support (like silica or alumina), the column is called a *bonded column*. In HPLC, the diameter of the particles that make up the column's packing material is proportional to the constant C described in the *Van Deemter* equation.

The columns are prone to accumulation of sample matrix and other impurities in the head area and such effects may lead to the undesired effects in elution, including peak broadening, split peaks etc. However, before a column is considered as unfit for any further use, analysts prefer to regenerate it. 'Column regeneration' is one method of cleaning the column and making it fit for a limited use further. The regeneration protocols are specifically provided by column manufacturers. Ultra High Performance Liquid Chromatography (UHPLC) columns are generally not recommended to be regenerated. The HPLC columns can be regenerated by disconnecting the column and connecting the outlet of the column to the pump. This reverses the flow direction of solvent within the column and facilitates cleaning.

In measures of protecting the column and the LC system from damage, one can consider use of 'guard columns'. Guard columns are connected in between the injector and the analytical column and they provide protection from entry of impurities from sample into the column. It is recommended to use a guard column of the same material as that of the analytical column. Guard columns are available in two major types: cartridge type and the packed type.

Cartridge guard columns (size ranges commercially available are 3mm to 10 mm) are easy to install compared to the packed guard column (size ranges commercially available are 3mm to 10 mm). The use of an in-line filter in addition to guard column enhances the protection provided to the column and the system against impurities.

- ***Mobile Phase Reservoir and Filtering***

The solvents for HPLC are generally stored in glass bottles. Commercially such glass bottles are available with specially fabricated caps, tubings made up of Teflon and filters that connect to the inlet of pump and purge gas (helium) that is used to remove dissolved gases. The two possible points from where the dissolved gases in a solvent can enter the instrument are the suction end of a pump and the column outlet that is connected to a detector. An interruption can be caused by an air bubble that can block the flow through a column. This problem mainly arises in aqueous solvents which have a higher solubility for gases especially when there is a gradient process and the water/organic ratio keeps changing. Conventionally dissolved gases are removed by degassing by ultra sonication for 5-10 mins, or vaccum for 5-10 mins or sparge (purge) the solvent with a gas that has a very low solubility compared to the oxygen and nitrogen from the atmosphere. Helium is the generally preferred solvent for degassing as it has low solubility in water, and its solubility is less affected by temperature. It is advisable to apply vaccum for 5-10 min and then store under Helium atmosphere for degassing aqueous solvents.

- ***Sample Injection***

Sample introduction can be done through an injection valve or through fully automated automatic sampling devices which operate with the help of autosamplers and microprocessors. Liquid samples can be directly injected for analysis and solid samples are dissolved in solvents, preferably mobile phase to avoid the interferences caused by detector with other solvents. All the samples to be injected should be free from particulate matter which can be removed by filtering over a 5 µm filter.

- ***Pumps***

A HPLC pump is used to push the solvent and sample through the column. The variation in elution process can be reduced by maintaining a constant, pulse free, flow rate by the pump.

Multi-piston pumps offer such features as it is equipped with two pistons, out of which one controls the flow rate and the other recharges. *Syringe pumps* offer a good control of flow rate; however, the only drawback of syringe pumps is that they are unable to produce as much pressure as piston pumps.

- **Detectors**

The detector is situated at the end of the column, to detect all the components. One cannot generalize a particular detector for all types of separations. Most commonly used detector is a UV absorption detector, as most of the molecules absorb UV radiation. Fluorescence and refractive index detectors are also used for special applications. The latest type of detectors been introduced are the NMR detectors which allow detection and quantitation of components by nuclear magnetic resonance after the separation process.

Optical detectors are used most commonly in HPLC systems. Such a detector passes a beam of light through the flowing column effluent as it passes through a low volume (~10 µl) flow cell. The change in the output voltage is affected by variations in light intensity caused by UV absorption, fluorescence emission or change in refractive index, from the sample components passing through the cell. The resultant voltage changes are recorded on a strip chart recorder and are processed by a computer to provide retention time and peak area data.

Apart from UV detector the other commonly used detectors are Photo Diode Array UV detector (PAD), refractive index(RI), fluorescence (FLU), and electrochemical (EC). The RI detector is also called as universal detector but has less sensitivity. The fluorescence and electrochemical detectors are very selective and sensitive (upto 10-15 pmole concentrations).

- **Data Systems**

Using modern data collection techniques, the analysis of the detector signal can be carried out. The data can be stored and retrieved later with the aid of sophisticated computer analysis. The main aim of using electronic data systems is to increase the accuracy and precision of analysis, without any operator assistance. If highly automated analysis systems are not available one can use a pre-programmed computing integrator for data analysis. When higher control levels are required, intelligent processors can be used. The automation options are easier to implement and analysis of complex data becomes more feasible. The advanced analysis options assist in optimization of chromatographic runs and deconvolution (i.e. resolution) of overlapping peaks. The software also helps in maintaining confidentiality of data by providing user specific options.

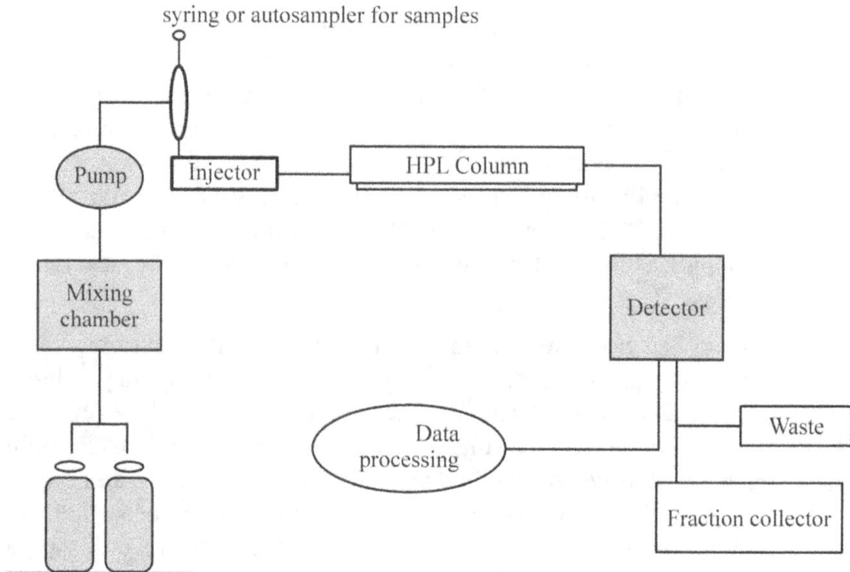

Figure 6.1 Diagrammatic representation of HPLC unit

Types of HPLC Techniques

Normal Phase vs. Reverse Phase

In normal phase HPLC separations, the stationary phase is more polar than the mobile phase, whereas in reverse phase the stationary phase is less polar than the mobile phase. In reverse phase HPLC the polar compounds elute faster and non-polar compounds are retained longer. The aim of a HPLC separation is to elute the components in as short time as possible, considering the optimum resolution. Thus, the determination of the appropriate ratio between polar and non-polar components in the mobile phase becomes a critical factor for efficient separation. The goal is for all the compounds to elute in as short a time as possible, while still allowing for the resolution of individual peaks. Normal phase columns are packed with alumina or silica and reverse phase columns contain alkyl, aliphatic or phenyl bonded phases.

Gradient Elution vs. Isocratic Elution

In an isocratic elution the composition of the mobile phase is kept constant throughout the analysis. When a sample contains components of a wide range of polarities a gradient chromatography, is the technique of choice. In this technique, the ratio of polar to non-polar compounds in the mobile phase is kept on changing. In a reverse phase gradient, the solvent composition starts with relatively polar and slowly becomes more non-polar. The gradient elution has the benefits of providing complete separation of all the peaks, without taking an excessive amount of time. The only limitation is that it requires more complex and expensive equipment and it difficult to maintain a constant flow rate in gradient flow. At high speeds, gradient elution will make results less reproducible and prone to variation. When the flow rate or mobile phase composition varies even slightly it affects the reproducibility of the results.

Application in Hyphenated Techniques

HPLC can be applied for qualitative and quantitative determinations. Most of the separations today are carried out by reverse phase technique. Reverse phase HPLC (RPLC) becomes ineffective when substances like inorganic ions, polysaccharides, polynucleotides need to be analyzed. Substances like amines, sugars, lipids, amino acids, peptides, proteins and pharmaceutically active compounds are easily separated by RPLC.

One can exploit the advantages of chromatographic techniques through hyphenated techniques which combine spectral methods to chromatography. Data regarding the chemical components present in a mixture is obtained from chromatographic technique and information regarding the identification of components using standards or library spectra can be obtained from Spectroscopy. About two decades ago, Hirschfeldcoined the word "hyphenation", which means an on-line combination of a chromatographic technique for separation and one or more spectroscopic techniques for detection. A diagrammatic representation of hyphenated technique instrumentation is given in Figure 6.2.

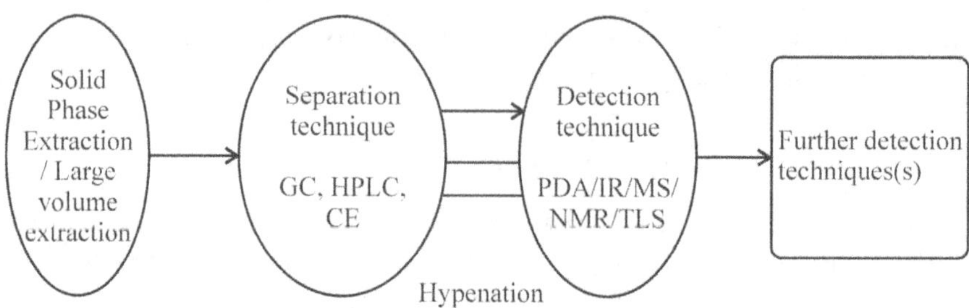

Figure 6.2 Hyphenated technique instrumentation

Hyphenated techniques have gained increasing importance as the technique with both quantitative and qualitative analysis features can solve complex analytical problems.

A Chromatographic technique like gas chromatography (GC), liquid chromatography (LC), high-performance liquid chromatography (HPLC), or capillary electrophoresis (CE) is linked to spectroscopic detection techniques, like photodiode array (PDA) UV-vis absorbance or fluorescence emission, Fourier-transform infrared (FTIR), nuclear magnetic resonance spectroscopy (NMR), and mass spectroscopy (MS) for obtaining structural information and identification of the compounds present in sample. These combinations have led to the introduction of hyphenated techniques, like GC-MS, CE-MS, LC-NMR and LC-MS. HPLC and MS or NMR in hyphenation is applied to the analysis and structural determination of complex phytoconstituents. LC-MS is used more than LC-NMR in many applications due to its attributes of better sensitivity in detection. The hyphenation of techniques can be between more than two techniques for example LCPDA-NMR-MS, LC-MS-MS, LC-PDA-MS, LC-NMR-MS. When analysis involves the detection of trace amounts of substances, the instrumentation may involve combination of solid-phase extraction (SPE), large volume injection (LVI) or solid-phase microextraction like LVI-GC-MS or SPE-LC-MS.

Hyphenated techniques also provide the advantage of having excellent separation efficiency and obtaining on-line complementary spectroscopic data on an LC or GC peak of interest in a complex sample. This chapter provides an overview of basic instrumentation principles of modern hyphenated techniques.

Liquid Chromatography-Infrared Analysis (LC-IR)

The coupling of an LC technique with infrared spectrometry (IR) is called as LC-IR or HPLC-IR hyphenated technique. HPLC is one of the most widely used separation technique and FTIR helps in the identification of particular functional groups in organic compounds. The hyphenation of HPLC and IR is difficult and is a slow process. This is because in the hyphenation with IR, the absorption bands of the mobile phase solvent are quite large and the identification of small signals of the sample analyte becomes difficult.

The limitations of IR technique are overcome by the recent advancements in HPLC-IR technology viz., the *flow-cell approach* and *solvent-elimination approach*. In the flow cell approach used with LC-IR the technique is identical to the one used in UV-vis and other LC detectors.

In the *flow cell approach*, an interference is introduced by the absorption of the mobile phase, however in the mid-IR region the transparent region can help in some detections. If during analysis, a mobile phase consisting of a deuterated solvent is used (for example heavy water or perdeuterated methanol), then IR can easily examine the organic compounds that have C-H structures in the molecules.

In the *solvent-elimination approach*, the mobile phase solvent is removed and IR detection is carried out in a medium that is transparent for IR light. Salts of KBr or KCl are used to collect sample components in the eluent, and then the medium is heated before the IR detection eliminates the volatile solvents in the mobile phase. Diffuse-reflectance infrared Fourier transform (DRIFT) approach and buffer-memory technique are two methods that are used for elimination of solvents. Now-a-days units having the interface for GC, HPLC, and SFC hyphenation along with IR technique are also available. A diagrammatic representation of HPLC- IR hyphenated system is shown in Fig. 6.3.

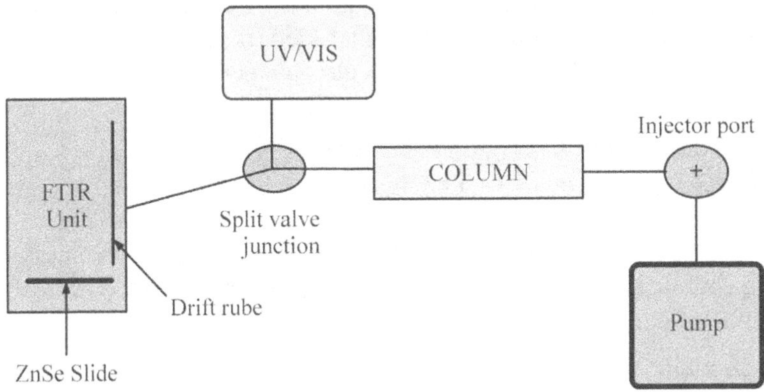

Figure 6.3 Diagrammatic representation of HPLC- IR hyphenated system

Liquid Chromatography - Mass Spectrometery (LC-MS)

LC-MS or HPLC-MS refers to the coupling of an LC with a mass spectrometer (MS) where the sample that is eluted from the column after separation is identified based on its mass spectral data. With an autosampler, an LC system, and the mass spectrometer, an automated LC-MS system has a double three-way diverter in-line where the diverter operates as an automatic switching valve and it diverts the undesired portions of the eluate from the switching valve to waste before it is introduced into the MS. Diagrammatic representation of HPLC-MS hyphenated system is shown in Fig. 6.4.

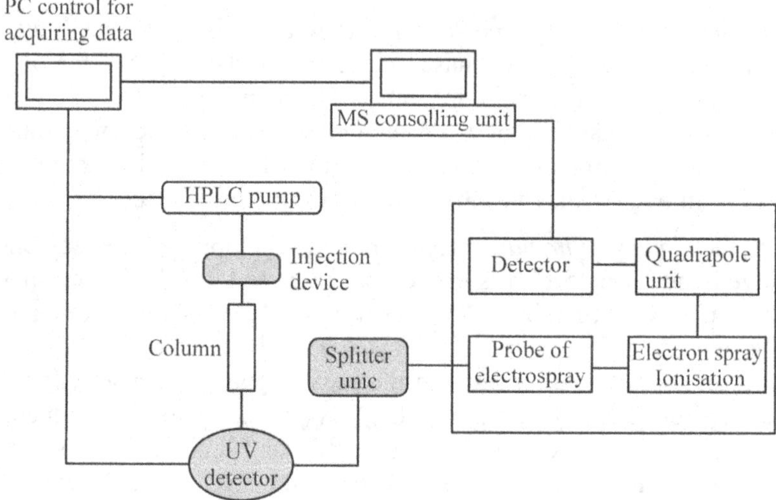

Figure 6.4 Diagrammatic representation of HPLC- MS hyphenated system

The combination of LC and MS helps in chemical separation of an analyte and the confirmation of its molecular identity. The data about the fragmentation pattern of the analyte molecule obtained from MS analysis helps in confirming the identities of compounds.

The data obtained from a single LC-MS run is comparatively poor and often requires introduction of Tandem mass spectrometry (MS-MS) to get more detailed information from fragments through collision-induced dissociation of the molecular ions produced. Hyphenated techniques involving coupling of HPLC to UV and mass spectrometry (LC-UV-MS) have been used extensively for biological screening of herbal products.

Commercially various types of LC-MS systems with varying types of interfaces are available, the most widely been used are the electrospray ionization (ESI) and atmospheric pressure chemical ionization (APCI)

units. The interfaces are assembled in a way that they provide sufficient nebulization and vaporization of the solvent, elimination of the surplus solvent vapors, sample ionisation, and extraction of ions in the mass analyzer.

In LC-MS analysis, an analyst would prefer a reversed-phase system using a gradient or isocratic solvent mixture of water, Acetonitrile, or methanol to which mobile phase modifiers like acetic acid, ammonium acetate, or formic acid may be added. In combination with these interfaces, different types of analyzers, like ion trap, quadrupole, or TOF, can be used.

LC-MS systems do not give the analyst a complete and definite on-line identification of components, unless the component is well-known and that its complementary on-line spectroscopic information is available in the databases. One of the major drawbacks associated with LC-MS is that the quality of response depends on many factors, like the nature of the analytes, the mobile phase composition, the type of interface used and the flow rate. Optimization of the ionization conditions that can be suitable for different types of compounds is a very difficult process; hence it is advisable to analyze the extract in different ionization modes.

Liquid Chromatography - Nuclear Magnetic Resonance (LC-NMR)

NMR is considered to be one of the least sensitive methods among the various spectroscopic techniques available to date. The first on-line HPLC-NMR coupled analysis was carried out using super conducting magnets in the early 1980s. With advancements in technology the coupling of HPLC systems to NMR, gave rise to the new techniques of HPLC-NMR or LC-NMR. LC-NMR is used widely in the analysis of complex mixtures especially samples of natural or herbal origin and metabolite analysis of biofluids.

LC-NMR experiments can be carried out in various flow methods like the continuous-flow and stop-flow modes. The vital requirements for on-line LC-NMR, apart from the NMR and HPLC instrumentation, are the continuous-flow probe and a valve that helps in recording the NMR spectra. The detector used in LC operation is a UV-vis type. For HPLC-NMR coupling magnetic field strengths higher than 9.4 T are recommended. Many bioanalytical experiments can be carried out using 500, 600, and 800 MHz systems with 1H, 2H, 13C, 19F, and 31P probes.

The construction of analytical flow cell was done initially for continuous-flow acquisition, but with increasing demand for complete structural assignment of unknown compounds application in the stopped-flow mode was carried out.

The construction of stopped-flow modes was promoted by the benefits of the closed-loop separation-identification circuit, along with the advantages offered by the 2D and 3D NMR techniques with complete automation. A typical representation of LC-NMR is shown in Fig. 6.5.

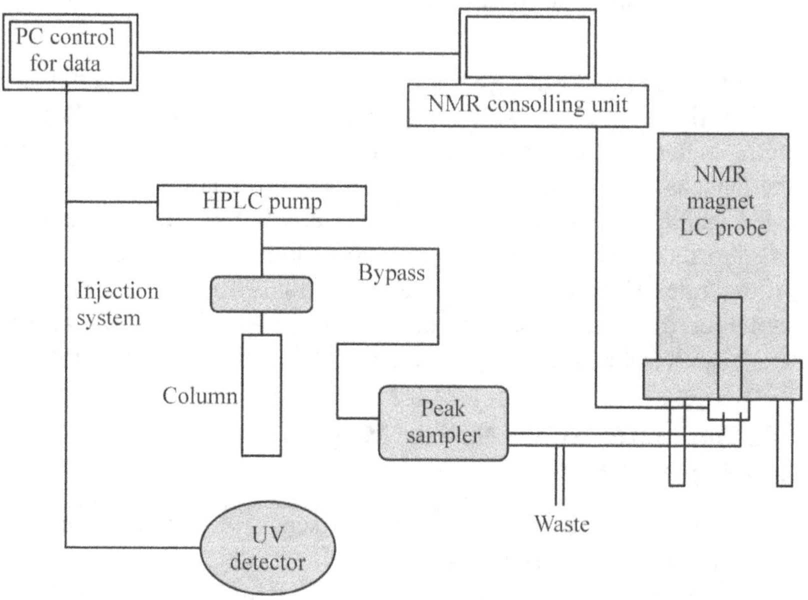

Figure 6.5 A typical representation of LC-NMR system

In a typical LC-NMR system, the LC unit consists of an autosampler, the pump, column, and a non-NMR detector (like DAD, UV, refractive index, or EC). From the detector, the flow of eluent is directed to the interface of LC-NMR. The interface can be set with supplementary loops for the intermediary storage of LC peaks of interest. From the interface the flow is then directed either towards the flow-cell NMR probe-head or towards the waste collector. After passing through the probe-head, the flow is directed to a fraction collector. The collected fractions can later be utilized for recovery and additional studies of the various fractions analyzed by NMR. The entire unit can also be attached to a MS via a splitter at the output of the LC-NMR interface.

During a LC-NMR operation, reversed-phase columns are used and they utilize a binary or tertiary solvent mixture with isocratic or gradient elution method. The protons in the solvents used may pose hindrance in obtaining an adequate NMR spectrum. The receiver of the NMR spectrometer is unable to differentiate between the strong solvent signals and the weak substance signals simultaneously. This drawback is overcome by solvent signal suppression that is attained by soft-pulse multiple irradiation or pre-saturation. This difficulty can also be reduced by using solvents (such as methanol, acetonitrile or water) that have as few 1H NMR resonances as possible, using atleast one deuterated solvent (like D_2O, ACN-d_3 or MeOD) in the mobile phase composition, using ionpair reagents that have as few 1H NMR resonances as possible and using buffers with very few 1H NMR resonances as possible (e.g. ammonium acetate or TFA).

As compared to other hyphenated techniques, the sensitivity of LC-NMR is very less and thus it is necessary to develop a suitable LC separation method that can help the analyst to obtain a concentrated quantity of the separated compound with the least elution volume. LC-NMR is a complementary technique to LC-UV-MS with a potential for further applications in detailed on-line structural analysis. With the latest developments in NMR technology a new impulse to LC-NMR is gained, and it is upcoming as a powerful analytical tool. Recent progresses in the coupling of hardwares and softwares of hyphenated instruments have brought about the automation of the entire process. The advancements include; flow-cell design, new systems for several solvent suppression and capability of automatic peak-picking and storing. The technique of HPLC-NMR has been used in many areas like analysis of herbal products, detection of organic molecules, biological samples, analysis of drug impurities and by-products, chemical reaction mixtures, and degradation products of drugs. For the analysis of natural products, HPLC-NMR is been combined with a many homo and heteronuclear 2D NMR analyses like the 2D total correlation spectroscopy (TOCSY) or 2D nuclear Over hauser enhancement spectroscopy (NOESY). However, due to its low sensitivity in detection and high operation cost, LC-NMR has not been widely accepted as compared to other hyphenated techniques. The recent developments in the field of chromatographic science, with respect to the advancements in pulse field gradients and solvent suppression methods, the development in probe technology, and the establishment of high-field magnets (800-900 MHz) have presented new momentum to this technique.

Capillary Electrophoresis - Mass Spectrometry (CE-MS)

The technique of Capillary Electrophoresis was introduced in the early 1990s. Capillary Electrophoresis with the help of electric field helps in separation of many substances of varying nature. This feature of CE, becomes an advantage to the versatility of this method. In this method the separation occurs by application of voltage across capillaries filled with buffer, and the separating ions then move at varying speeds after the application of voltage, based upon their size and charge. The peaks of solutes are observed as they pass through the detector and the quantitative determination of peaks is carried out. Diagrammatic representation of a typical CE-MS system is shown in Fig. 6.6. When the unit of CE is attached to a MS for acquiring on-line MS data of the analyte, the resultant arrangement is termed as CE-MS.

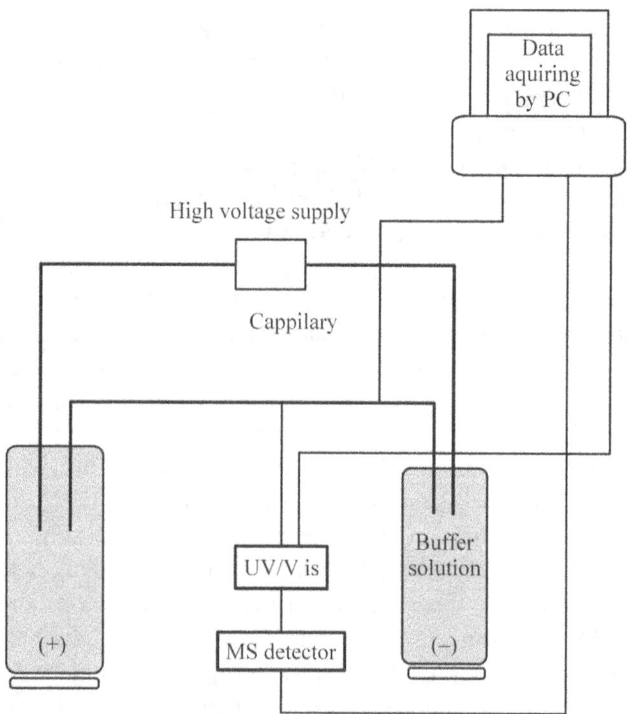

Figure 6.6 Diagrammatic representation of a typical CE-MS system

Separation occurs through the channels etched on the surface of the capillary through which the sample is delivered to Electro spray Ionization Mass Spectrometer (ESIMS). The instrumentation is completely automatic and it has a high degree of sensitivity and selectivity. Another type of interface known as *coaxial sheath liquid CE-MS interface* that was developed recently, allows the use of both LC-MS and CE-MS in an alternate manner on the same mass spectrometer. A sheath liquid passes via the pump and avoids the flow of any current towards the ground. The alternative shifting between LC-MS and CE-MS modes can be done in minutes. In order to avoid the electrical problems, the power supply from CE is used to provide potential for both, CE separation and the ESI sprayer tip. The technique of ESIMS detection is used widely for the analysis of biomolecules, herbal products, and characterization of analytes based upon their molecular weight and structures. However, the interfacing of CE with MS is a challenge as CE requires low flow rates, and which can be achieved only by incorporation of a make-up liquid.

7 Gas Chromatography and Mass Spectrometry

Introduction

The *gas chromatography* (GC) or *gas-liquid chromatography* (GLC) technique is a form of partition chromatography in which the mobile phase is composed of a gas and the stationary phase is a liquid. A test substance is injected into the gas phase where it is volatilized and is passed onto the liquid phase. It is then held in some form in the column. Analytes spend varying times in the mobile phase and the stationary phase, depending on their comparative affinities for the stationary phase. The peaks then elute from the end of the column exhibiting peaks of varying concentration, like a Gaussian distribution. These peaks are detected by a detector and passed onto a recorder, and an integrator, so that the progress of the chromatographic separation can be observed and quantified.

The technique was first brought into focus in the 1950s and since then it has been subjected to continuous development in aspect and progress is still being made. Till 1980s, the potential of the technique was not readily accepted as it had disadvantages like their high cost, a limited durability; and substantial losses of polyunsaturated components from the walls of the columns available commercially in that decade. The development of columns in the later years entirely discarded all these disadvantages.

Theoretical Aspects and Instrumentation

- *Few Basic Considerations*

  A basic gas chromatograph has three essential components, i.e. some form of inlet through which the sample is introduced onto the column, the column itself which contains the stationary (liquid) phase and through which the mobile (gas) phase is passed continuously, and a detector. The column is the principal component of concern, and there are three main types of it. In the initial years of inception of GC instrumentation, the main unit of work of gas chromatography was a packed column, made up of a glass or metal tube, about 2 - 4 mm in internal diameter and 1.5- 2.5 m in length. It was coiled to fit the oven unit and was filled with an inert solid support coated with the liquid phase. Support-coated open-tubular (SCOT) columns are made up of a narrow bore tubing (0.5 to 1.25 mm i.d. in lengths of 10 to 15 m) and they consist of a powdered solid support coated with a liquid phase. Wall-coated open-tubular (WCOT) columns consist of narrow bore tubing (0.1 to 0.3 mm i.d. and 25 or 50 m in length commonly), of glass or fused silica, which is coated with the liquid phase on the inner walls. A conventional packed column is packed with the liquid phase on its particulate support. Conventional packed columns are rugged in use and can handle large sizes of samples and their resolution is limited. WCOT columns offer excellent resolution, but the parameters like size of the sample and the method of its introduction are decisive.

The column allows partitioning of the constituents of the sample to be separated between the stationary and mobile phases, and this is supported by the liquid phase been available as a thin film with a large surface area to the gas phase. As the sample moves down the column, the molecules of each component partition themselves sandwiched between the liquid and gas phases. As the gas phase moves continuously, the solute molecules get dissolved in more and more of the liquid phase, they resurface into the gas phase and pass further down the column.

As long as a molecule is in the gas phase, it travels down the column at the same speed as the carrier gas. When a mixture of sample is in the solute, the components diffuse into the liquid phase according to their individual equilibrium constants, and move down the column at varying rates. It indicates that their retention times on the column are different and the components tend to separate based upon their retention times. The component particles are irregular in shape and size and the liquid phase will also comprise of regions of different depths. In a WCOT column, there is only a single flow path and the liquid phase is usually more uniform in thickness, thus the factors that lead to band broadening are minimized. Components emerging from packed columns are wide bands compared to the time spent on the column, while those rising from a WCOT column are comparatively narrow. Thus, the efficiency of a column relies upon on the degree of band broadening which is imposed upon a solute when it passes through a column in a given period of time. The shape of the concentration peak of a component is controlled by band broadening (width) and its absolute concentration in the gas phase. Under conditions of constant temperature, the distribution constant/coefficient (K_D) remains unchanged and the efficiency of a given column can be related to peak widths and retention times. Along with many practical issues, however, it is necessary to increase the column temperature during an analysis in order to bring off less volatile solutes in a rational time, and then the calculation of column can be carried.

Under isothermal conditions when solutes separate in accordance with their equilibrium constants, peaks would appear with a Gaussian distribution. Column efficiencies are then calculated in terms of numbers of theoretical plates (n), the retention time (t_r) measured from the point of injection until the peak reaches its maximum, and the width of the peak measured at half its maximum height (w_h) by using the equation:

$$n = 5.54 \times (t_r/w_h)^2$$

The units used to measure t_r and w_h must be same. These parameters are exemplified in Fig. 7.1. Column efficiencies may be expressed in terms of theoretical plates per metre, or according to the column length (plate height) comparable to a single theoretical plate. Preferably, retention volumes rather than retention times must be used, although both the terms are apparently related in a given column.

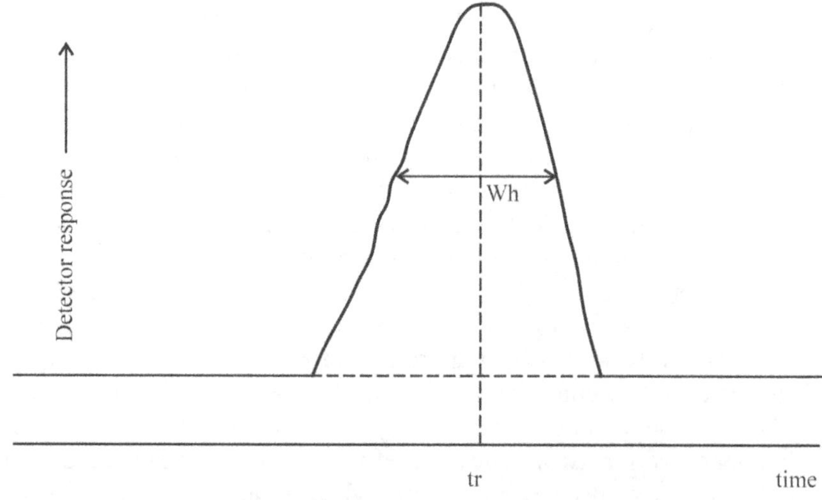

Figure 7.1 A chromatographic peak with an ideal Gaussian shape

Calculation of the Efficiency of a Column

For a component that does not dissolve in the liquid phase, a particular volume of gas which is required to carry it through the column, and this is volume of gas which is termed as the hold-up volume. It is easier to calculate hold-up time (t_m) rather that hold up volume. This is generally measured by injection of methane onto the column and determination of the time for the emergence of the foremost edge of the methane peak. If every solute molecule spends similar hold-up time (t_m) in the gas phase, the true time spent in the liquid phase is therefore an adjusted retention time (t^1), that can be calculated as:

$$t^1 = t_r - t_m$$

The quality of the separation should not be affected by the time spent by the components in the gas phase. Compared to packed columns t_m is relatively great in WCOT columns. The true efficiency in terms of *effective theoretical plates* (N) is calculated as:

$$N = 5.54 \times (t^1/w_h)^2$$

The ratio of the weight of the solute in the liquid phase to the weight in the gas phase, is termed the *partition* or *capacity ratio* (k), and it is proportional to the time spent by the solute in the liquid phase and the gas phase, i.e.

$$k = t^1/t_m$$

The major differences between packed and WCOT columns are based upon the relative availability of the liquid and gas phases to a solute molecule, and this can be defined as the *phase ratio*, β , i.e.

$$\beta = \frac{\text{Volume of gas phase}}{\text{Volume of liquid phase}}$$

and in fundamental nature in a WCOT column it can be defined as

$$\beta = r_o/2d_f$$

where r_o - the radius of the capillary

               d_f - the mean depth of the liquid film

Consideration of Practical Inferences

The efficiency of a column depends upon a number of factors, like the column dimensions, nature and flow-rate of the carrier gas, liquid-phase thickness and column temperature. By optimizing these factors, a considerable resolution can be achieved. Whereas, improved resolution may also be brought about at the cost of an increased analysis time. Practically, it is desirable to select parameters for an analysis that give adequate resolution in a reasonable time.

The primary factors in selection of a carrier gas are its nature and velocity. At high velocities, the chances for band broadening are reduced, but there may then be inadequate time for them to pass through the liquid phase. Conversely, when the flow-rate of the mobile phase is low, there are more chances for band broadening. Therefore, efficiency is liable to be affected in both the conditions. The selection of the carrier gas is also important. For example, hydrogen and helium (especially hydrogen), has a high diffusivity (low resistance to mass transfer) are greatly to be preferred to nitrogen. It is also worth mentioning that column efficiency varies much less with gas velocity over the working range when hydrogen is used. Thus, a précised calibration of flow is less decisive in practice.

If hydrogen is used as the carrier gas, it is necessary to safeguard the working against the risk of explosions, for example through ignition of leaked gas byan electrical spark. With increase in temperature during temperature-programming, there is a decrease in the efficiency of the columns. The components emerge as sharper peaks, as the vapor pressure of the solute rises.The flow-rate through the column decreases with increased temperature as the viscosity of the gas is increased. Thus, a temperature-programmed analysis should preferably be initiated at a higher gas velocity than might be used for an isothermal run. This effect tends to be in a reduced amount with hydrogen than with other carrier gases.

The column length, column internal diameter and film thicknessare the three factors which are dependent on the physical characteristics of the column. Out of these above mentioned factors, column length is least important as it can be known that resolution is proportional only to the square root of column length. Thus, if one has to improve by a factor of two on the resolution to be achieved with a 25 m column, it would be essential to move to one 100 m in length, and this would predictably mean that the analysis time would be increased by a factor of four.

In distinction by reference to the last equation above, it is evident that changes in the column internal diameter or in the film thickness will have a marked effect on the partition ratio. If the column diameter is reduced, it leads to a decrease in the phase ratio and a proportional increase in the capacity ratio can be obtained. The overall analysis time and retention times of solutes are increased. A decrease in film thickness will correspond to an increase in the phase ratio and thus lead to a decrease in the partition ratio. Practically, the nature of the solute must also be taken in to account, for solutes of high volatility films with higher thickness must be preferred.

Carrier Gas

The carrier gas plays an important role in GC analysis. The carrier gas to be used for analysis should be dry, free of oxygen and chemically inert. Helium has a larger range of flow rates, is safer than hydrogen, and is compatible with many detectors. Other gases like nitrogen, argon, and hydrogen are also used depending upon the desired performance and the detector being used. Hydrogen and helium are commonly used in Flame Ionization (FID), thermal conductivity (TCD) and Electron capture (ECD). Both these gases provide a shorter analysis time and lower elution temperatures of the sample due to higher flow rates and low molecular weight. Mass spectroscopy detectors use nitrogen or argon gases as carriers and have higher molecular weights, which thus improve vacuum pump efficiency.

Carrier gasses are commercially supplied in pressurized tanks with pressure regulators, gauges and flow meters to monitor the flow rate of the gas. Ideally the gases available should have purity range between 99.995% - 99.9995% and must contain low levels (< 0.5 ppm) of oxygen and total hydrocarbons.

Column Oven

The temperature of the column is controlled by a thermostat oven (as shown in Fig. 7.2. The oven can be operated in two manners: isothermal programming or temperature programming.

In the temperature programming the temperature of the column is gradually increased at rates of 5-7 °C/minute. This type of temperature control helps in separating a mixture with a broad boiling point range as it detects low boiling point components and high boiling point components as the analysis proceeds slowly towards rising temperature.

In an isothermal programming, the temperature of the column is held constant throughout analysis. Thus, at a lower temperature low boiling fractions are well resolved but the high boiling fractions are slow to elute. And, at a higher temperature the higher boiling components elute as sharp peaks but the lower boiling components elute so fast that they are not separated.

Columns

- ### *Packed Columns*

  Since the time the technique of gas chromatography was first developed, Packed columns have been in use. Analysts used stainless steel columns for many years, and now the most preferred columns are the glass columns as they are almost inert, permit visualization of the column packing conditions (gaps in filling, deterioration of packing material at the inlet end etc.) and they can be easily emptied for reuse. The only drawback is that they are relatively fragile, and need special care during handling.

  The solid supporting materials for the liquid phases are usually diatomaceous earths, (usually 80-100 or 100-120 mesh), and can be deactivated by washing with acid and by silylation in order to increase the life of the liquid phase and to reduce any adsorptive effects on the solutes. Supporting materials that are pre-coated with liquid phases are also available commercially. One can prepare his own supporting material by filtering the liquid phase through a bed of the support and then whole material can be dried in form of layers; the amount of liquid phase that is left back on the support can be then determined. Satisfactory coatings can be obtained by coating the liquid phase on the support and evaporating in a rotary evaporator flask. This process helps in protecting the surface of the support against any damage. A column can be packed by adding the coated support material with a funnel, and applying a vacuum to the exit end. After filling, a glass wool plug (acid-washed and silanized) should be placed on top of the packing. The column can be conditioned for about 48 hours at a temperature slightly above the highest temperature at which it is to be operated during routine analyses, before been put in use. A well-packed column (1.5 to 2 m) that contains a support with 10-15% (w/w) of the liquid phase should exhibit an efficiency of 3000 to 5000 theoretical plates. Care must be taken that if columns are too tightly packed, they are blocked or the injection syringes may get plugged and if they are too loosely packed, they result into very poor separations.

- ***Glass WCOT Columns***

Analysts took about some years to be convinced about the robustness of Glass WCOT columns for routine use in the laboratory. The glass columns offer good resolutions and have inert surfaces. The interests of analysts for glass columns increased when glass drawing machines for capillary production became available commercially at reasonable cost. The surface of the glass columns are treated chemically to ensure adhesion of a liquid phase. This is because surface tension in the liquid may cause it to form droplets and leave the surface of the glass. Gaseous etching or aqueous leaching treatments are preferred methods of treatment of glass columns. Wetting agents, carbonisation and silylation, were used before the advent of etching and leaching techniques for treating glass columns. The pretreatment process with such agents helps in increasing the contact angle between the glass and liquid phase, as small pores or crevices on glass are filled with the agents and they help in spreading of the liquid film. The etching process also scrupulously cleans the glass surface, and the chemical treatment can alter the surface so that the liquid film is deposited on salt crystals and not on silica particles. Borosilicate glasses such as Pyrex™ are treated with HF gas, where the silicate structure is attacked to form silicon tetrafluoride, which forms crystals covering the surface. Soda glass is treated with HCl, the reaction is extremely complex and involves a preliminary leaching of alkali metals from the surface and needs deactivation before coating of liquids. Care should be taken that a new WCOT column must be conditioned before use.

Glass capillary columns have the disadvantage of fragile nature, and requires utmost care when columns are mounted in or are removed from the oven of the gas chromatograph. The column ends must be straightened before the column can be fixed in place, and this process requires some skill and practice.

- ***Fused Silica WCOT Columns***

Fused silica columns consist of an amorphous silicate material, free of metal oxides. The material is inert and has proved to be an excellent medium for the manufacture of WCOT columns. These columns are very flexible and thus they overcome the disadvantage of glass columns of straightening the ends. They are covered on the exterior with a polymeric material which avoids fragile fractures. The liquid phase is bonded chemically to the surface by various means and the individual molecules of polymeric liquid phases are cross-linked by chemical methods to enhance their stability at elevated temperatures. Organic impurities from the stationary phase can be removed by passing a little solvent through it. These advantages of fused silica columns have increased their importance in comparison to glass columns.

The Liquid Phase

- *Selectivity*

  The basic requirements of a stationary phase are to provide reasonable chemical and thermal stability, and a proper degree of selectivity for the separation. The selectivity of a liquid phase depends upon various factors, and must be determined experimentally. It can be accomplished by comparing the retention times of various test substances. The polarity of the liquid phase is a major factor that influences separation according to the degree of unsaturation. When only packed columns were established the polarity of liquid phase, was a rather variable property, because of the variations in the loading of the liquid phase, the nature of the solid support, and the different operating factors such as temperature and column age. The problems could not be absolutely eliminated even after improvements in the production of liquid phases.

- *Increasing Column Life*

  The stationary phase on a column can deteriorate due to many reasons, but generally occurs due to chemical attack. As WCOT columns contain less stationary phase, they are more prone to deterioration than the packed columns. Polar solvents like alcohols and minute amounts of polar impurities in the columns can react slowly with the liquid phase and may deteriorate the column when exposed to excessive temperatures. Polar liquid phases have a tendency to react with oxygen or water molecules are thus care must be taken that the carrier gas is free of these and suitable molecular sieves and oxygen scrubbers should be placed between the gas cylinder and the column to avoid them. The carrier gas flow should not be stopped as long as the column is being heated. Also, due to the change in characteristics of liquid phase, non-volatile materials injected onto a column tend to get accumulated over a period of time. If the damage to column has occurred in the initial few coils, a particular length of it can be broken off without affecting the column performance. Sometimes if the damage is minimal the column can be reversed and used.

Effects of Matrix

While performing an analysis one has to deal with various aspects of a sample, especially a batch of samples that have a range of physico-chemical properties and if they have to be analyzed in a single run. Sometimes in an analysis procedure the residues of matrix co-extracts inevitably pass through into the prepared purified sample.

The detector and injector sites may face interferences due to such interfering matrices and may lead to errors in quantification, ruggedness, and analyte detectability.

The fundamental approaches that an analyst may apply to overcome the matrix assisted errors are to improve quality assurance by eliminating primary causes of these errors, optimizing the calibration approach (internal standard or standard addition method) and injection and separation parameters.

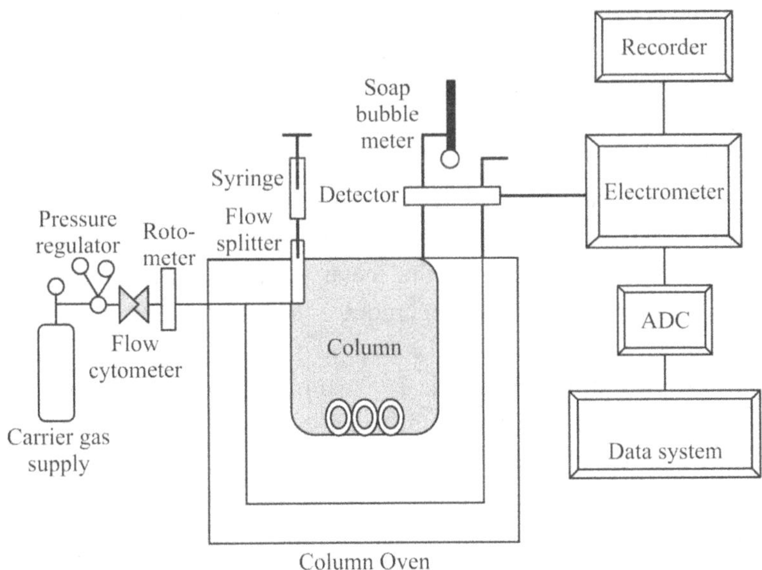

Figure 7.2 GC Instrumentation

Injection Systems

There are various types of inlet systems for GC, viz. split/splitless, cold on-column injector, and programmed temperature vaporiser.

Certain factors inhibit the reproducibility of results in trace analysis of foods. Below mentioned are some undesirable effects which may occur during food analysis and are associated to the type of injection systems used:

(i)   change in the composition of sample,

(ii) poor reproducibility of the amount of sample and retention times,

(iii) thermal degradation, adsorption, rearrangement, of analyte and

(iv) impairment of separation

The strategy to be adopted for introduction of sample depends upon various factors like concentration range ofintendedanalytes, their physico-chemicalproperties and amount of matrix extracts present in the sample.

An important aspect to be considered is that during the injection process the sample should not change in composition, (thermal degradation if occurs should be negligible). The column efficiency should not be lost, there should not be any interference caused to the detection of the solutes by the solvent peaks, and the retention times and peak areas should be highly reproducible. Not only the instrumentation, but all the other factors of injection technique should be carefully considered. The difficulty of volatilization which occurs due to early evaporation of the sample before the needle is completely inserted into the injector or when the sample is in contact with the metal surface of the needle can be minimized. The **"hot needle"** technique is suggested for such problems. In this technique, the sample (0.1 to 1 μL) is drawn up totally into the syringe barrel, and the needle is kept empty. The needle is introduced firmly into the injection port, and it is allowed to warm up for about 5 seconds before the plunger is pressed rapidly.

Some analysts also prefer to use **"solvent flush"** method. This method is similar to **hot needle** method, the only difference being that a small plug of fresh solvent is drawn up ahead of the sample, and is used to push the sample into the evaporation chamber.

There are many types of injection systems for WCOT columns as explained below:

- ***Split / Split Less Injection***

  WCOT columns may often be overloaded due to a large volume of sample as their capacities are very limited. To overcome this problem, many injection systems have been developed. A diagram of such a split/split less injector is shown in Fig. 7.3.

  In the **"Split Injection"** method the sample is volatilized in the carrier gas. This mixed stream is then divided into two parts, one of which moves towards the column and the second is let out to the atmosphere. The flow through the vent towards the atmosphere is regulated before injection by a control valve to give the preferred split ratio, (about 1:20 to 1:200). Due to the high flow rate in the column (1 to 2 ml/min), the gas flow through the injector is very high (100 to 200 ml/min) and the vaporized sample stays in the injector only for a very short duration of time. After introduction of the sample, the carrier gas passes into the column. The vaporization chamber has a glass or quartz liner that provides an inert surface vaporization. The demerit of this injector is that it may differentiate against the higher boiling components of a sample, and the quantification can be erratic. When the sample size is small, this type of injection cannot be used as much of the sample is wasted.

  For most advantageous analysis, the nature of the solvent and its volume should be kept constant, the initial column temperature should be obtained accurately like the previous one and the syringe needle should always enter to the same spot above the column inlet.

  A **"Cold Trapping"** technique can also be used during injection. In cold trapping method the column temperature is upheld at the boiling point of the solvent; and as soon as the sample re-condenses as a narrow band, and the solvent peak is observed to appear, the oven is heated up rapidly to the normal analysis temperature. This cold trapping utility is nowadays available in commercial gas chromatographs and can be carried out automatically.

  In the **"Split Less Injection"** method the *"Solvent Effect"* is applied. In this type of injection mode, the sample is injected in a solvent with a boiling point higher than the column temperature and allowed to pass in a chamber where only the carrier gas for the column flows. After an optimized time period, about 1.5 times that is required for the carrier gas to sweep out the injection chamber, a purge valve is opened. The gas is allowed to flow towards to the bottom of the inlet. The gas flow then gets divided into two streams, out of which one stream continues as the carrier gas while the second stream takes away any residual sample from the injection chamber. A schematic representation of a typical split/splitless injection system, which can be used in either mode, is shown in Fig. 7.3. The technique has most value in the analysis of trace components.

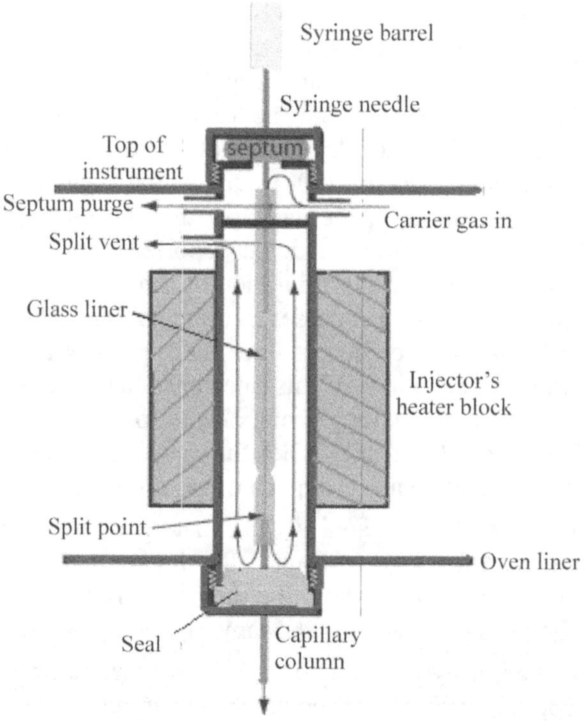

Figure 7.3 Diagram of a typical split/splitless injection for WCOT GC columns

- ***Cold On-column Injection (COC)***

   In a cold on-column injection, the sample is injected onto the column directly with a solvent. The temperature of the column is maintained near the boiling point of the solvent and the sample is concentrated by **"Cold Trapping"** or a **"Solvent Effect"**. The column inlet has a soft elastomer **"Duck-bill"** valve, which consists of two plastic surfaces pressed together by the pressure of the carrier gas in the injection port. When the injection is done, a needle of fused silica is slipped between the two surfaces and is directed into the top of the column.

Such an injection method causes less thermal degradation of analytes. Further enhancement in features can be attained by changing the polarity of column stationary phase, or decreasing its diameter and thickness to permit fast analysis at lower temperatures.

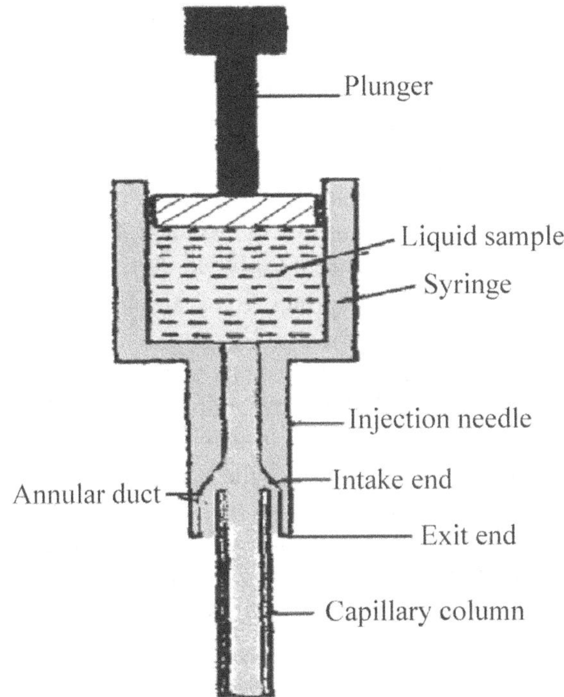

Figure 7.4 Cold On-column injection construction

- ***Programmable Temperature Vaporization (PTV) Injection***

Programmed-temperature injection also known as PTV is based upon the split or splitless mode of injection. At the moment of injection, the injector chamber/inlet is cool. As soon as the sample is introduced into this inlet, the temperature is increased at a controlled rate so that the sample components are vaporized in a selective way.

This type of injection is suited for thermo labile components and analytes with a broad boiling range. As the liner size can be increased in PTV, it is more suitable for on line coupling and trace analysis of analytes. PTV methods are compatible with various capillary columns including the columns with a narrow bore.

Detectors

An ideal GC detector is expected to have the following characteristics, although not a single detector can meet all the requirements together. The detector should possess adequate sensitivity and give a high resolution signal for all components. The detectors should be chemically inert and should not change the sample in any way during analysis. Furthermore, they should be reliable, predictable and easy to operate.

- ***Flame Ionization Detectors (FID)***

  The flame ionization detector is widely accepted and used due to its attributes of having high sensitivity and stability, a fast response time, a low dead volume, and having an extremely wide range for linearity. FIDs are simple in construction and operation, (see Fig. 7.5) and are reliable in extended use.

  The detector works on a principle of combustion of the organic compounds in a diffusion flame of hydrogen and air, as they emerge from the column. The carrier gas can also be mixed with hydrogen gas. The outlet of the column is generally situated at the orifice of the combustion jet. The collector electrode is constructed above the flame, and a potential between the collector and the jet opening is established, thus enabling the measurement of ion current. A potential is selected in the saturation region to prevent the recombination of ions. The amplifier receives the signal current that matches with the calibration of the detector and is then transmitted to a recorder.

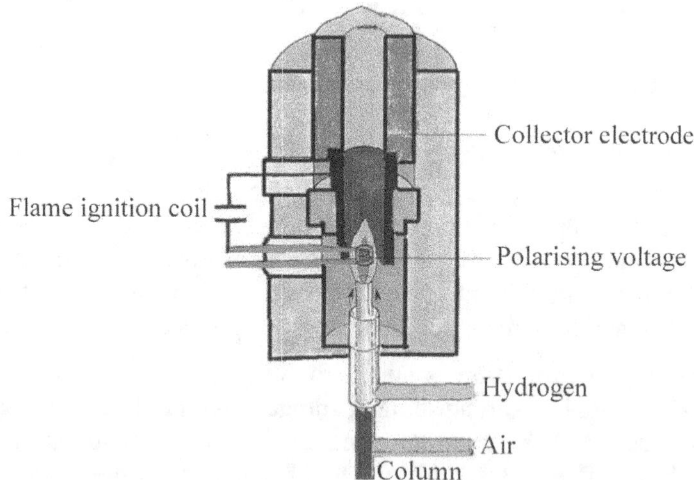

Figure 7.5 Representation of a flame ionization detector

- ***Electron-Capture Detectors (ECD)***

  In the electron-capture detector (Fig. 7.6), the carrier gas is bombarded with β particles (from a radioactive source) and it is passed on to the ionisation chamber. The β particles generate up thermal electrons (each β particle generating thousands of electrons) to a thousand, which are collected by applying a voltage potential. When the solutes containing electron-capturing moieties are introduced into the cell, a decrease in the background current is observed due to the interaction of the solute and the thermal electrons. This background current can then be measured with a high sensitivity.

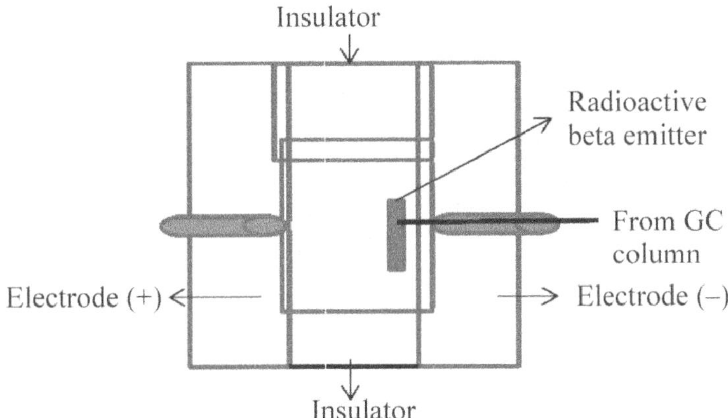

Figure 7.6 Electron capture detectors

- ***Thermal Conductivity Detectors (TCD)***

  Thermal conductivity detectors (TCD) are one of the oldest detectors used with gas chromatography. The presence of the sample causes a change in carrier gas thermal conductivity and this is measured by a TCD (Fig. 7.7). The construction of a TCD is relatively simple, and it is made up of an electrically heated source that is maintained at constant power. The temperature of the source (platinum or gold) is dependent upon the thermal conductivities of the surrounding gases. The resistance of the wire is affected by the thermal conductivity of the gas which is responsible for the temperature rise.

  TCDs make use of a pair of detectors, one of which monitors the thermal conductivity of the carrier gas and sample mixture and the second one is used as the reference for the carrier gas. Carrier gases such as helium and hydrogen have the advantage that due to their high thermal conductivities even a small amount of sample is readily detected.

The TCDs have the advantage of being easy and simple in use, the recovery of analyte can be done after separation and detection and its utility in detecting wide range of compounds from inorganic to organic nature. The biggest drawback of the TCD is the low sensitivity of the instrument in comparison to other detection methods.

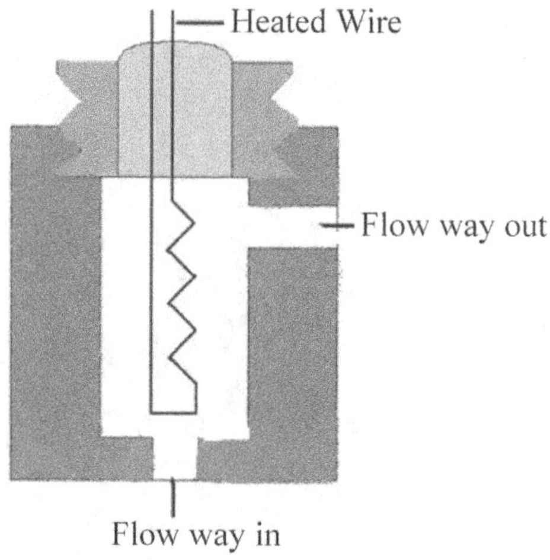

Figure 7.7 A Thermal conductivity detector cell

- ***Atomic Emission Detectors***

  Atomic emission detectors (AED), are the latest form of detectors used for GC. These detectors utilize a partially ionized gas (plasma) to atomize all of the elements of a sample and excite their characteristic atomic emission spectra. These detectors are based on the detection of atomic emissions and thus have a wider applicability. The detectors generate plasma by three ways: microwave-induced plasma (MIP), inductively coupled plasma (ICP) or direct current plasma (DCP). MIP is the most commonly used form and it monitors the atomic emission spectra of several elements due to a positionable diode array (Fig. 7.8).

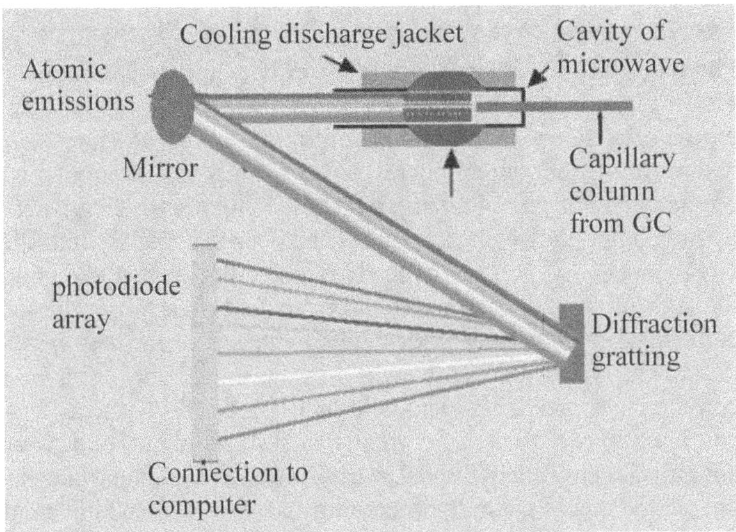

Figure 7.8 Representation of an Atomic emission detector

- ***GC Chemiluminescence Detectors***

  Chemiluminescence spectroscopy (CS) utilizes the optical emission from excited chemical species for determination of both qualitative and quantitative properties. It utilizes the light emitted from the energized molecules rather than just excited molecules like an AES detector (Fig. 7.9). AES detectors are designed for gaseous phases whereas chemiluminescence can occur either in the solution or gas phase. The light energy is obtained from the reactions of the chemicals and this light band is used as a substitute to a separate light source.

  CS has the limitation that it requires a photomultiplier tube (PMT) which utilizes a dark current to detect the light emitted from the analyte.

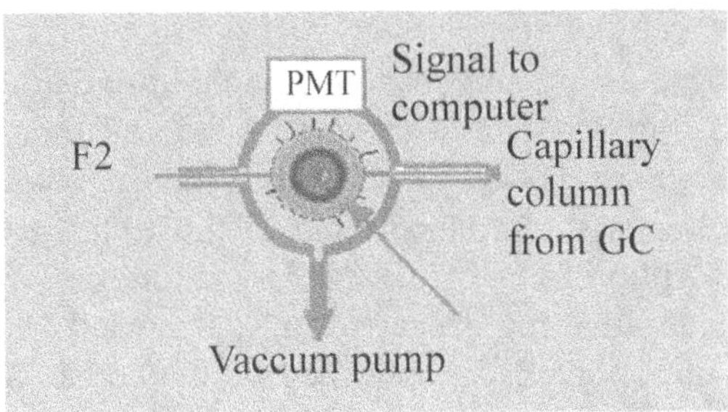

Figure 7.9 Representation of a GC chemiluminescence detector

- ***Photoionization Detectors***

  Photoionization detector (PID) is a detector which applies the properties of chemiluminescence spectroscopy for detection. PID enables the selective estimation of aromatic hydrocarbons, organo-hetero atom, inorganic species and other organic compounds. PID consists of an ultraviolet lamp that emits photons which are absorbed by the compounds in an ionization chamber that has an outlet from a GC column (Fig. 7.10). The analyte molecules in small fractions are ionized in a non-destructive manner and this property enables confirmation of results with detection been performed with other detectors. Immediate analysis results can be obtained by commercially available hand-held models of PIDs with various lamp configurations. PID is used greatly in soil, sediment, and water and airanalysis. However, the PIDs have the disadvantage that they are unable to detect certain hydrocarbons like methane and ethane due to their low molecular weights. PIDs are not suitable for detection of semi-volatile compounds, and they require frequent calibration during working. The rapid variation in temperature at the detector affects instrumental signal obtained during analysis.

- ***Injection by use of Microvials***

  The technique of injection of samples by use of disposable micro-vials is also called as Direct Sample Introduction (DSI) or Difficult matrix introduction (DMI). In this type of sample injection technique the liner system is equipped with a disposable micro-vial which has been placed in it. It helps in analysis of large volumes of samples, where only volatile and semi-volatile compounds are excluded into the GC system during thermal desorption process and the non-volatile sample matrix is retained on the wall of microvial. The various types of commercially available micro-vials are depicted in Fig. 7.11.

- ***Solid-phase Microextraction (SPME)***

  This technique uses a solvent free sample introduction technique. A fused-silica fibre is coated on the outer side of the stationary phase. From the headspace or by direct immersion the volatile analytes get extracted directly and concentrated to the fibre coating after their thermal desorption in the heated GC injection port. This method has the advantage that the process can be carried out with a fully automated option available, and the liner and column do not require maintenance. This sample introduction technique employs use of strong matrix effects, thus problems in quantification may arise.

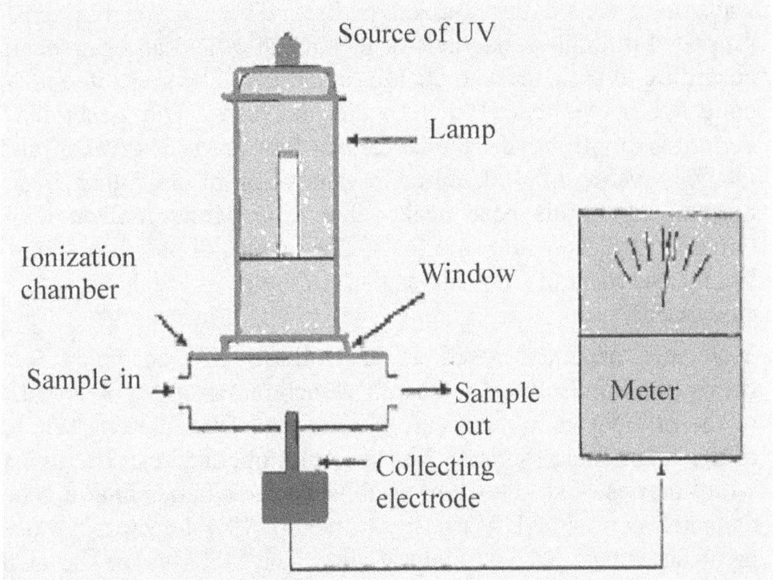

Figure 7.10 Diagrammatic representation of a photoionization detector

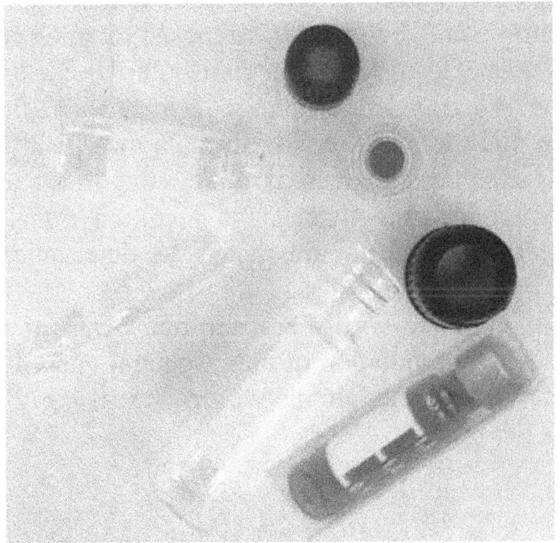

Figure 7.11 Commercially available vials for GC

• *Mass Spectrometry Detectors*

The basic principle of this method is that organic molecules in the vapour phase, form positively charged ions when they are bombarded with electrons. These charged ions fragment in various ways to give smaller ionized entities. These generated ions are propelled through a magnetic or electrostatic field and get separated according to their mass to charge (m/z) ratio. The generated ions are collected in sequence as the ratio increases. The generated ion current is amplified and the largest (or base) peak is given a random intensity value of 100, and the intensities of the other ions are normalized to this base peak value. The parent molecule ion is termed as the *molecular ion* (M^+). The masses of individual ions can be measured and the molecular formula of each ion can be calculated.

Molecules fragment based on the splitting that occurs at weaker bonds (the bondsclosest to specific functional groups). The structure of the original compound can be estimated from the characteristics of the fragments produced. The spectrum obtained can be compared with libraries of structures of established compounds until a good fit or match is obtained. Mass Spectrometer (MS) detectors are one of great advantage to GC analysis. In a GC/MS system, the analyte masses are scanned continuously by a mass spectrometer till the separation step. After passing through the column when the sample exits, it is passed through a transfer line into the inlet of the mass spectrometer. The sample is exposed to an electron-impact ion source where electrons ionize the molecules by causing them to lose an electron due to electrostatic repulsion. Thus, the sample gets fragmented and the ions are passed into a mass analyzer where they are sorted based upon their m/z or m/e value (mass to charge ratio). The GC chromatogram depicts the retention times and the mass spectrometer will analyze the peaks to determine the nature of molecules in the mixture. The figure below represents a typical mass spectrum of n-octane with the absorption peaks at the appropriate m/e ratios. The combination of mass spectral and GC retention data help to remove any other alternative structures.

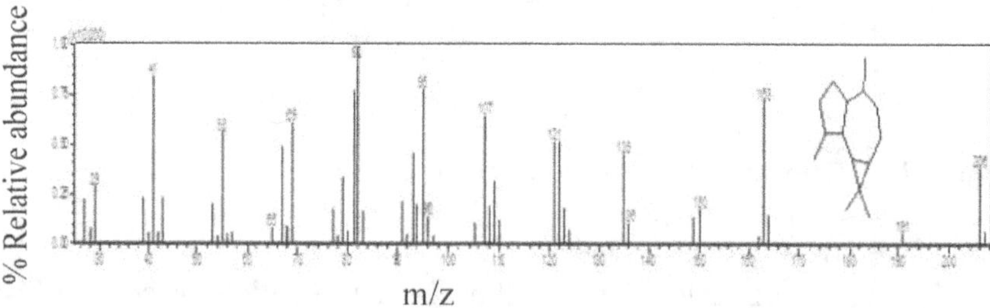

Figure 7.12 A typical mass spectrum

When a gas chromatograph is interfaced with a mass spectrometer, a basic condition is that the pressure must be reduced from column (atmospheric pressure) to the ion source (10^{-4} torr). The interface must be as inert in nature and the occurrence of *cold spots* (spots where sample condenses) should be eliminated. The extra-column volume should be as little as achievable to reduce band broadening. Recently, the advent of fused silica capillaries has made these issues simpler to be dealt with. A new range of diffusion pumps with the capacity to withdraw helium at the same rate as it comes out from a column are available. Also, Teflon membrane or molecular jet separators are available to concentrate the solute relative to the carrier gas.

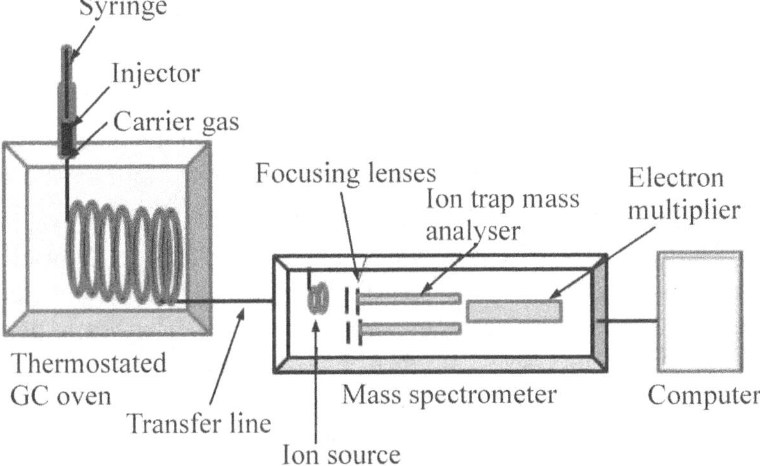

Figure 7.13 Diagrammatic representation of the GC/MS system

The advantages of GC/MS units are that they allow simultaneous determination of the mass of the analyte, identification of target analyte and components of incomplete separations. The GC/MS instruments are rugged, and easy to use. One of the major disadvantages of mass spectrometry detectors are that samples may thermally degrade before detection and ultimately the results may be affected.

Mass Analysers In GC

The selection of a good mass analyser depends on many factors such as physico-chemical properties of analytes, nature of matrix, target analyte properties, cost of instrumentation, through put demands *etc.* that must be considered. There are various types of mass analyzers available and some of them are described briefly below:

- *"Quadrupole Ion-trap Analyzers"* are one of the most common types of mass analyzer in GC/MS. They hold gaseous anions or cations for long periods of time by electric and magnetic fields. A simple quadrupole ion-trap analyzer can use a ***full scan mode*** for operation or a **selected ion monitoring** (SIM) type of mode. A hollow electrode will be constructed such that ions can flow into the cavity. A variable radio-frequency can be applied to the electrode and ions with an appropriate m/z value will orbit around the cavity. With a linear increase in the radio-frequency, ions of a stable m/z value are ejected based upon their mass. Too heavy and too light ions are destabilized and neutralized upon collision with the electrode wall. When the ejected ions strike on the electron multiplier an electrical signal is generated. With the help of various soft wares, this electrical signal is then converted into data that can be interpreted to estimate the characteristics of a sample.

- *"Time-of-flight Mass Analyzers"* (TOF) measure the flight time of samples in a field free tube sample molecules. The neutral molecules are used to generate gaseous ions which are accelerated to produce constant kinetic energy and then ejected into a mass analyser by use of electric-field gradient oriented towards the ion beam. The generated electric field gradient has a positive influence on mass resolution of the instrument. The improvement in mass resolution is brought about by using reflectron (ion mirror). Ions with a higher energy pass more deeply inside in the reflectron area and the extent of time until the time they reflect back is noted. As a result, the ions of the same mass to charge ratio strike the detector approximately at the same time. The times of flight of the separated ions are proportional to the square root of respective m/z value. The TOF-MS instruments use a multi channel plate (MPC) detector for analysis. There are various types of accessories like time-to-digital converter (TDC), analogue-to-digital (ADC)-based continuous averager, also called digital signal averager (DSA) or integrating transient recorder (ITR) that a TOF-MS instrument uses for analysing TOF of ions. Such features have helped in developing instruments with high-resolution analysers featured with only moderate acquisition speed, and unit-resolution instruments that have a high acquisition speed.

- ***Instruments with Double-focusing Magnetic Sectors***

  Single sector magnetic mass analyzers operate by using only a magnetic field to separate ions based upon their mass to charge ratios. With the help of an electric field the ions entering the mass analyser are accelerated and only ions with a particular charge are passed through a magnetic field. Depending on their mass the charged ions tend to move in a circular path in amagnetic field and reach the ion detector at varying locations.

  In contrast to the *single sector magnetic mass analyzers,* the *double sector mass analysers* are equipped with an additional electric field that only filters ions with a particular kinetic energy and are then passed through to the magnetic sector. The ions are then separated based upon their mass in the magnetic sector as in the routine process.

- ***Tandem Mass Spectrometry***

  Tandem mass spectrometry (MS/MS) involves the application of at least two stages of mass analysis, in combination with a dissociation process or a chemical reaction that brings about achange in the mass or charge of ions. Fundamentally, there are two different advancements in MS/MS operation. The first one is *'in space'* method, in which two physically distinct parts of instruments are coupled together (*e.g.* triple quadrupole, QqQ). The second type is *'in time'* in which a sequence of events in an ion storage device are performed (*e.g.* ion trap, IT).

  Product ion, precursor ion, neutral loss, selected reaction monitoring, multiple reaction monitoring, and MSn scans are the most important tandem MS/MS scan modes. MS/MS methods generally engage the activation of ions by collision with an inert gas which leads to fragmentation.

  - The ***precursor ion scan*** method selects the ion of interest, activates and carries out mass analysis of the product ions.

  - The ***product ion scan*** method performs processes opposite to that of a precursor ion scan.

  - The ***neutral loss scan*** method involves scans for a neutral loss of fixed, predetermined mass.

  - In ***MSnscan*** method a precursor ion is selected and isolated by ejecting all other masses from the mass spectrometer. Collision-induced dissociation (CID) of the precursor ion generates ions with varying masses (MS/MS). Except for the product mass of an analyte the other fragment ions are expelled from the cell. The retained back product ion can then be, again subjected to CID, yielding more product ions that can be mass analysed (MS/MS/MS). Such a process canbe repeated a number of times.

- The *Selected reaction monitoring* (*SRM*) is a type of SIM. A tandem instrument is used to enhance the selectivity of such type of SIM.

- *Multiple reaction monitoring* (*MRM*) is used to examine several reactions in a process.

- The major benefit of using MS/MS is the intolerance against the chemical noise, which may be due to various factors like matrix compounds, column bleed, contamination from an ion source etc. Each MS-step directs some loss in intensity of the analyte signal, however it also gives the benefit of a greater loss in the noise, and thus there is an increase in S/N ratio.

Limitations of GC Analysis

- ***Response Factor:*** In order to obtain reproducible results of response factor, the analytical results should be considered as comparable only if the experimental conditions, including the detector are kept identical for a particular sample.

- ***Worn Septum:*** The septum of an injection port is affected adversely by temperature changes. A septum would last for a span of about 200 injections after which issues like leakage and deposition of samples on it may affect the sensitivity of the instrument.

- ***Injection Port Temperature***: If the temperature of the injection port is not appropriate it may lead to either poor separation (due to low temperature) or degradation of components (due to high temperature). This may ultimately result into interference of deposited substances with the analyte of interest during analysis.

- ***Residual Impurities***: Impurities that reside into the column and elute in the later analysis of other samples may lead to inappropriate results of the target samples.

- ***Carrier Gas***: The selection of carrier gas for analysis is an important task. The selected carrier gas should not be unstable or impure.

- *Operational Skills*: Only well skilled personnel should be allowed to operate the instrument as there are various factors like; method of injection, column temperature, gas flow rates, pressure etc. which need to be well monitored to sustain the performance of the instrument for a longer duration.

Limitations of Mass Spectrometry

- *Resolution*: A high resolution is best suited for MS analysis; low resolution does not yield appropriate data for interpretation.

- *Pressure*: MS analysis should not be performed under high pressures, when low pressures are used they advantageously reduce collisions.

- *Parent Mass*: Parent mass is determined based upon the parent peak. However, for high molecular mass compounds, identification becomes a difficult task. Chemical ionization MS, reduces the probability of missing the parent mass.

- *High Speed Scanning*: Rapid analysis of specimens can be carried out with *High speed scanning MS* instruments. However, increased speed reduces the resolution of peaks.

- *Technician's Skills*: A technician's skill and proficiency in determining the molecular structure from mass spectra patterns is required in addition to the computer assisted database analysis.

- *Crucial Factors*: MS has a highly sensitive instrumentation and utmost care should be taken about trace of a sample remaining in the instrument and affecting further analysis. All the analysis should be performed in comparison to a suitable standard obtained for particular sample types.

Limitations GC-MS

- A contamination due to impure carrier gas may occur in analysis.

- If GC step of analysis does not occur in an appropriate way, it will lead to erranious MS feed and increase in "Background noise".

- The analytical evidences should always be established after careful verification with another reliable technique.

Applications

- Gas chromatography is used widely in separation and identification of volatile organic compounds that include metabolites generated by specific bacteria after infecting food samples, phyto-pesticides in vegetables, additives added in sauces, beverages and meat products.

- It is used in analysis of herbal and pharmaceutical formulations containing volatile oils, cosmetic formulations, human saliva, breathe and blood containing volatile organic substances.

- With GC coupled with FID the components like Polycyclic aromatic hydrocarbons (PAHs) in air samples can be analyzed. Due to the higher concentrations of PAHs in the environmental samples GC–MS operated in SIM mode represents appropriate technique for their determination.

- Semi volatile food toxicant compounds, like pesticides can be analysed by GC–MS.

- Industrial contaminants like Polychlorinated biphenyls (PCBs) enter the food cycle through various human activities. GC equipped with ECD or MS detector can be used for analysis of such compounds.

- Industrial processes used for manufacturing plastics, textiles, furnishing foams lead to incorporation of chemicals like polybrominated diphenyl ethers (PBDEs) which can be analysed with GC techniques.

- The detection of mycotoxins can be carried out by derivatisation with trimethyl silyl ethers and the perfluoro-esters.

- Various veterinary drugs used for therapeutic treatment of animals can be determined for their presence in meat and other animal by-products like milk etc.

8   Ion Exchange Chromatography

Introduction

Ion chromatography (IC) is a technique used for the estimation and separation of ionic solutes from samples. This chromatographic technique finds its application in environmental analysis, analysis of samples from industrial wastes, biological analysis, samples from pharmaceuticals and food products. In an IC analysis method, the liquid passes through a solid stationary phase that is porous in nature and the solutes are eluted into a flow-through detector. The stationary phase is composed of uniformly sized particles (of diameter 5-10 mm), packed into a cylindrical column. The material used for construction of column is either stainless steel or plastic and the internal diameter of it is 4-9 mm with length about 5-30 cm. With the aid of a high pressure pump the mobile phase is forced through the column at with flow rates of about 1-2 ml/min. The sample to be analyzed is injected into the solvent system with the help of an injection unit that is built before the column for manual or automatic injection depending upon the user preferences. The mobile phase carrying the sample passes through a small cell that is situated in the detector.

The basic instrumentation components for Ion chromatography (IC) are similar to that of HPLC, except for the chemistry of components that affects the separation and analysis of ions. Various types of solutes like inorganic ions, in organic cations, organic acids, and organic bases are analyzed by this technique. There are various chromatographic methods that are based upon separation the mechanism mentioned above (viz. Ion-exchange chromatography, Ion-exclusion chromatography, Ion-pair/ Ion-interaction chromatography and Capillary electrophoresis). However this chapter will focus upon Ion-exchange chromatography (IEC).

Principle of Separation in Ion Exchange Chromatography

The mechanism of separation by ion exchange chromatography is based upon the ionic interaction between the stationary phase and the sample or mobile phase carrying the sample. The stationary phase is charged with ions (cations or anions) which are neutralized by counter ions (present in mobile phase) that possess a charge opposite to the stationary phase ions. Ions from mobile phase or from the sample are exchanged by the counter ions and this is how the process of ion exchange chromatography occurs. During the process of Ion exchange, the electro neutrality of the solution is expected to be maintained and this would be attained when there is a stoichiometric exchange of the ions (i.e., a single anion displacing a single counter ion).

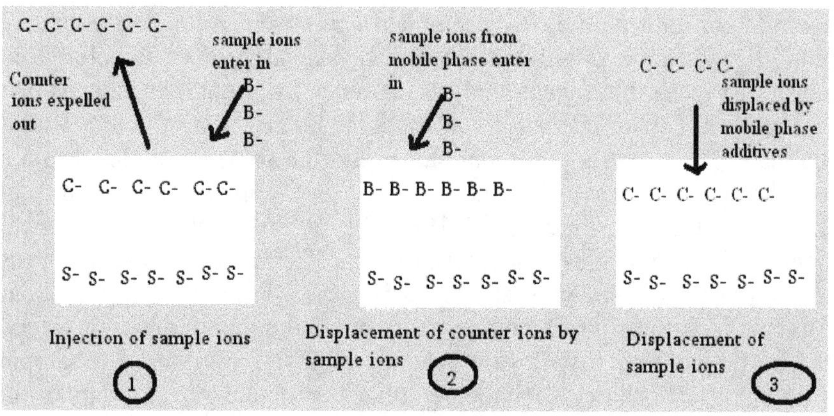

Figure 8.1 Diagrammatic representation of retention of ions in Ion exchange chromatography

- ***Stationary phases used in ion exchange chromatography***

  The Ion-exchangers in IEC are characterized by the type of the matrix of the stationary phase and the characteristics of the ionic groups present on the surface. There are two types of functional groups of exchangers commonly used in ion chromatography.

  1. ***Cation Exchangers:*** The examples of cation exchangers are; Carboxylic acid -COO^-H^+, Sulfonic acid -$SO3^-$ H^+, Phosphinic acid HPO^{2-} H^+, Phosphonic acid PO^3H^+, Phenolic -O^-H^+, Selenonic -SeO^{3-} H^+, Arsonic -$HAsO^{3-}$ H^+.

  2. ***Anion Exchangers:*** The examples of anion exchangers are; Tertiary amine -$NH(CH_3)^{2+}OH^-$, Quaternary amine -$N(CH_3)_2$ $(EtOH)^+$ OH^-, Quaternary amine -$N(CH_3)^{3+}$ OH^-, Primary amine -NH^{3+} OH^-, Secondary amine -$NH_2(CH_3)^{2+}$ OH^-.

  Cation-exchangers are classified as strong acid and weak acid type of exchangers. The strong acidic functional group exchangers are ionized over a broader pH range, whereas the weak acidic functional groups are ionized over a narrow range of pH. Except for the Sulfonic acid exchangers which are strong acid types, the other exchangers mentioned above under the class of cation exchangers are weak. The pKa of the weak acidic functional group should be lower than its pH.

Like the cation exchangers, the anion-exchangers are also classified as strong base and weak base exchangers. The anion-exchangers with quaternary amine functional groups form strong exchangers, whereas the less substituted amines form weak exchangers. The strong base is functional over a wide range of pH, whereas the weak anion-exchangers are functional over a narrow pH range. Majority of the ion-chromatography separations are carried out with silica or polymeric ion exchangers using either strong anion-exchanger or strong cation exchanger. The representation of instrumentation for IEC is given in Fig. 8.2.

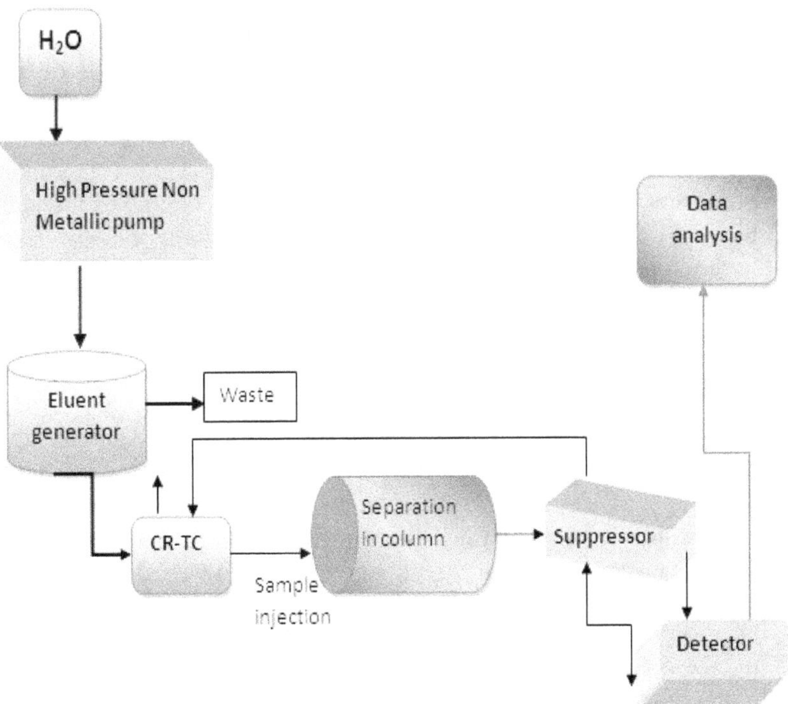

Figure 8.2 Instrumentation for Ion exchange chromatography

Matrixes

The matrixes that are used as support for stationary phases in ion chromatography are classified into three types as mentioned below:

1. ***Silica-based Materials:*** The silica-based stationary phases offer advantage of good efficiency, even under high pressures and stability. Silica-based stationary phases have disadvantages that they can be used only with pH range of pH> 2 and < 7 and the affinity to metal ions. The silica-based materials are either made up of functionalized silica, or the polymer-coated silica.

2. ***Synthetic Organic Polymers:*** These polymeric supports also commonly known as 'resins' are produced by synthesizing a polymer and then reacting it for introduction of ionic functional groups. These resins are tolerant towards the mobile phases with extreme pH values, ranging from 0-14. However, due to their relatively soft nature they are prone to limitations in pressure, with the exception of Macroporous (upto 1000 A) resins that are comparatively rigid and stable.

3. ***Hydrous Oxides:*** Minerals like alumina, aluminosilicates, or silica can be used as ion-exchangers and the excess charge of the matrix is neutralized by mobile counter ions. The metal oxide exhibit the feasibility of being used as cation- and anion-exchanger depending upon their acid or base properties. At lower pH values they exhibit properties of cation exchanger and can act as anion exchanger at high pH values. Thus, pH values form the selection criteria for hydrous oxide stationary phases.

Characteristics Affecting the Process of Ion Exchange Chromatography

1. ***Ion Capacity:*** The number of functional groups per unit weight of the stationary phase determines the ion capacity of ion-exchanger. The type of counter – ion available in the stationary phase is responsible for its swelling characteristics to a greater extent. Ion-exchange capacities of stationary phases have a vital role in resolving the concentrations of competing ions used in the solvent system for separation. While using higher capacity stationary phases, the conductometric detectors do not give a satisfactory performance due to the high concentrations of salts in mobile phase. For a typical ion-exchange process the ion exchange capacity is in the range of 10-100 mequiv/g.

2. *Swelling:* The ionic functional groups linked by polymer chains in organic stationary phases swell after coming in contact with water with swelling pressures of about 300 atmospheres. High ionic capacity and low cross linking are the characteristics advantageous to the process of swelling. The content of the mobile phase is very significant to the effect of swelling.

3. *Selectivity:* Depending upon the type of ion-exchanger and the conditions of use, there are variations observed with the relative affinities of different counter ions to the stationary phase. The extent of the ionic interactions are affected by some properties of the solute ions, the mobile phase ion and the counter ions like the charge on the solute ion, polarizing ability of solute ion, extent of cross-linking of ion-exchange polymers, size of the solvated ion, ion exchange capacity, and the type of functional group on the stationary phase.

The observed order of relative affinities of cations to strong acid cation exchange stationary phases are as follows:

$Pu^{4+} \gg La^{3+} > Ce^{3+} > Pr^{3+} > Eu^{3+} > Y^{3+} > Sc^{3+} >$

$Al^{3+} \gg Ba^{2+} > Pb^{2+} > Sr^{2+} > Ca^{2+} > Ni^{2+} > Cd^{2+} > Cu^{2+} > Co^{2+} > Zn^{2+} > Mg^{2+} > UO_2^{2+} \gg$

$Tl^+ > Ag^+ > Cs^+ > Rb^+ > K^+ > NH_4^+ > Na^+ > H^+ > Li^+ >$

For anions on strong base anion exchangers the order of relative affinity will be as

citrate$>$ salicylate$> ClO_4^- > SCN^- > I^- > S_2O_3^{2-} > WO_4^{2-} > MoO_4^{2-} > CrO_4^{2-} > SO_4^{2-} > SO_3^{2-} > HPO_4^{2-} > NO_3^- > Br^- > NO_2^- > CN^- > Cl^- > HCO_3^- > H_2PO_4^- > CH_3COO^- > IO_3^- > HCOO^- > BrO_3^- > ClO_3^- > F^- > OH^-$

It is difficult to provide very clear guidelines for control of separations, based only upon the data of degree of cross linking, and ion charges.

4. *Mobile Phases and their Properties for IEC:* By changing the ionic strength, pH or type of anions, the elution strength of the mobile phase can be controlled. The mobile phases used in IEC are generally made up of aqueous salt solutions and are classified based upon certain characteristics like: Suppressed or Non-suppressed compatibility with the detection mode, type of competing ion and its concentration, pH of mobile phase and its buffering capacity, ability of mobile phase to complex the ionic sample components and the organic modifiers used.

5. ***Compatibility with the Detection Mode – Suppressed or Non-Suppressed:*** The type of the mobile phase used for analysis is based upon the features of the detector used. The background signal (given by mobile phase) detected by the detector should not be too high. If there is no alternative to the use of such a mobile phase that provides high background signal due to its high conductivity in conductivity detector and highly absorbing in UV-VIS detector, a suppressor between the column outlet and the detector can be added to reduce the mobile phase interference.

6. ***Concentration and Nature of the Competing Ion:*** The mobile phase characteristics that influence solute retention are the affinities of the ions of sample and the competing ions of the mobile phase. When the mobile phase ions have a higher affinity to the stationary phase, the interactions of the sample ions and the stationary phase are reduced and thus result in lower retention times. The higher the concentration of the counter ions in the mobile phase the higher is the competition between the solute and the phase's ions and this leads to lowering of retention. Thus, the mobile phase should be selected by considering the appropriate charge, and effects of other factors like size, polarizability and concentration of salts in mobile phase to obtain a good separation.

7. ***pH, Buffering Capacity and Modifiers of Mobile Phases:*** The pH of mobile phase affects the charges on the mobile phase's ions, the solute ions and their ionization. The degree of protonation is increased with increase in pH and the mobile phase exhibits stronger elution properties. With an increase in the charge of the solute its affinity towards the functional groups on stationary phase increases and thus retention of solute increases. When pH independent ions are present in a mixture the pH of mobile phase becomes an important variable that can be altered to optimize separation. The buffering capacity of the mobile phase must be kept at a higher level to obtain better separations. For polyprotic solute ions' the change in pH can affect their retention and hence it is important to keep the pH of mobile phase constant. Some organic solvents that are water soluble (such as glycerol, acetonitrile, ethanol, methanol, and acetone) are added to the mobile phase for IEC separations. These modifiers affect the degree of complexation, and degree of ionization of ions in samples, mobile phase or stationary phase.

8. ***Metal Ion Complexation by Mobile Phase:*** Separations involving separations of metallic ions, are affected by the capacity of mobile

phase salts to complex them. Complexes are formed by the metal ion and the complexing agent and original charge and degree of ionization of the metal ion is changed. The new complex thus formed has a different retention times.

Ion-Suppression in Ion-Chromatography

The ion suppression is required in IEC when the mobile phase has a high conductivity and leads to a high background signal from the detector. In such cases, a tool, called the suppressor, is attached between the ion-exchange separator column and the detector. Upon attachment the device releases hydronium ions or hydroxyl ions based upon the nature of the mobile phase and corresponding non-ionized species are produced thus reducing their conductance. The suppressor enhances the conductance of solute and reduces the conductance of mobile phase and there is an improvement in the detectability of the solutes. A regenerant (or scavenger) solution is used to help the suppressor operate for extended period of time.

- *Solvent Systems (Mobile Phases/Eluents) used for Non-suppressed IEC*

  The solvent systems (mobile phases) for cations and anions vary considerably and few of them are listed below:

  Solvent systems for Anions: Aromatic carboxylic acids and their salts, Aliphatic carboxylic acids, Aromatic and aliphatic sulfonic acids, Potassium Hydroxide, Polyol-borate complexes, Ethylene diamine tetra acetic acid – EDTA, Inorganic Salts.

  Solvent systems for Cations: Inorganic acids, Organic bases

- *Solvent Systems (Mobile Phases/Eluents) used for Suppressed IEC*

  In the previous paragraphs, the functions of a suppressor are described. The suppressors help in the exchange of eluent cations for hydronium ions, where solvent systems with sodium salts of weak acids (carbonic, boric) are suitable. Suppressors help in exchange of eluent anions for hydroxide ions, where nitrate or chloride salts are appropriate. It also helps in eliminating the eluent ions completely by precipitation. Reduction of the charges of ions in the mobile phase is brought about by the suppressor by complexing them with complexantions like Cu^{2+}.

Detection Methods used in Ion Chromatography

The following detection methods are available with ion-exchange chromatography:

- ***Conductivity Detection***

  Conductivity detection has advantage of being universal in response, and its simplicity in construction and operation. The mobile phase that enters the detector is actually a conducting electrolyte. The electrical conductivity increases with increase in conduction by the solution. The conductance of a solution depends upon the ionic strength, temperature, and the specific conductance. When there is a significant difference in the ionic conductance of the solute and the mobile phase's ions a good detection occurs. A *direct type of detection* occurs when the conductance of mobile phase is low, and the entry of solute in detection cell causes an increase in conduction. And an *indirect type of detection* occurs when the mobile phase causes an increase in conductance and the entry of solute in detection cell causes a drop in conductance. Direct conductivity detection is applied in most IC methods for separation of anions and utilizes solvent systems containing organic bases. Indirect conductivity type of detection is used in separation of anions using hydroxide containing mobile phases and to for cations the mobile phase consisting of mineral acids.

- ***Atomic and Molecular Spectroscopic Methods***

  Spectroscopic methods are the most widely used methods of detection. Spectroscopic detection methods are of two types: molecular and atomic spectroscopy. Molecular spectroscopic methods comprise of methods like UV-VIS absorption, refractive index, fluorescence and phosphorescence. Atomic spectroscopy methods include techniques like flame atomic emission, flame atomic absorption, and plasma atomic emission.

- ***Electrochemical Detection***

  Electrochemical detectors are generally applied in tandem process along with a conductivity detector (that has the attributes of functioning more like a universal detector) and are applied in processes that demand more sensitivity and selectivity. The commonly used types of electrochemical detection are the Volta metric, Amperometric and coulometric methods.

- ***Detection by Post Column Reaction***

  This process involves the chemical reaction of the solutes when they are eluted from the column and just before they are introduced into the detector. This type of a step increases the selectivity and specificity of detector towards the solutes, even when there is a large interference from the matrix. Reagents like pyridine-2, 6-dicarboxylic acid, phenylfluorone, 2-(5-bromo-2-pyridylazo)-5-(diethylamino) phenol and ammonium molybdate, 4-(2-pyridylazo) resorcinol are used for post column reactions.

Applications of Ion Exchange Chromatography

- Ion exchange chromatography has in the separation of components and purification of many molecules such as antibiotics, vitamins, proteins, nucleotides, enzymes, DNA, and peptides from natural and plant products like *Nigella sativa* Linn., *Olea europea* L., hen eggs, *Phaseolus vulgaris*, dairy Whey, mulberry leaves, *Castanospermum austral, Paecilomyces variotii.*

- Ion exchange chromatography is applied in several processes in the manufacture of food and beverages, sugars and sweeteners, finishing procedures for metals, hydrometallurgy, analysis of chemical and petrochemicals, and analysis of softening of industrial water.

- Ion exchange chromatography is applied in removal of nitrates and natural organic matter from domestic water and production of soft water.

- Separation and chemical analysis of proteins, amino acids, DNA and RNA in biochemical studies are carried out by application of Ion exchange chromatography.

- Separation and purification of metals such as uranium, plutonium, actinides including samarium, lanthanum, neodymium, thorium, and lutetium. Analysis of other elements like hafnium and zirconium is also carried out with ion exchange chromatography.

- Ion exchange resins are employed in manufacture of redox batteries and fuel cells, removal of alkali from glass surfaces, and geo-technological processes that involve removal of pollutants from environment.

9   Chiral Chromatography

Introduction

The human body presents a very chiral nature at the cellular level. The activity of substances, their pharmacokinetics and pharmacodynamics is affected by their chirality. The first documented person to separate stereoisomers was Louis Pasteur. Pasteur, separated the stereoisomers by his observation that crystals of tartaric acid had two types: either left-handed or right handed crystals. He manually separated the two forms of crystals by using a microscope and tweezers. With the emerging facts about the problems caused due to stereoisomerism, researchers have focused their attention to enantio selective methods of separation and analysis. Literature reveals studies based on pharmacological and pharmaceutical properties of chiral drugs by using pre-column derivatization with chiral complexes, to form diastereomers. The formed diastereomers were separated with the help of normal or reversed phase mode of chromatography.

Stationary Phases

Since the last decade there have been significant contributions by researchers in developing better methods for enantioselective chromatographic process. Analysts have tailor made the stationary phases for chiral chromatography depending upon the type of analysis and nature of sample. Chiral stationary phases are preferred in analysis due to their advantageous attributes like, the speed of the analysis, utility in analyzing and purification of complex mixtures containing enantiomers, the reproducibility and flexibility of analysis. A schematic representation of chiral chromatography process is given in Fig. 9.1.

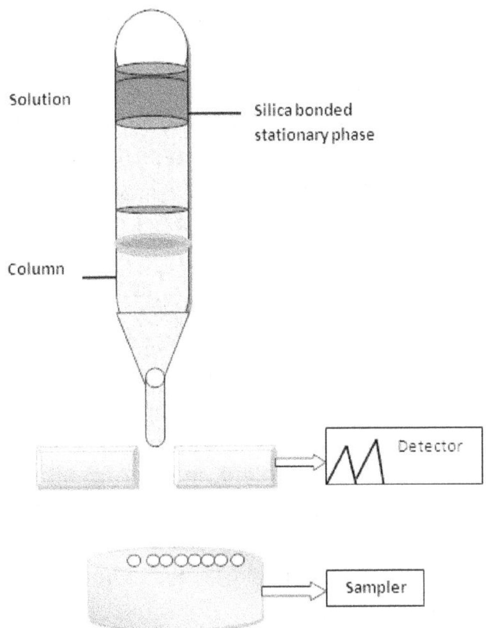

Figure 9.1 Chiral Chromatography analysis process

Chiral stationary phases are conventionally classified as below:

(i)   Ligand exchange (complexation of copper ions with chiral moieties).

(ii) Stereo selective contact to helical chiral polymers (the ones in derivatised form or available as free polysaccharides).

(iii) Steric interactions between chiral aromatic amide groups (with p-Donor and p-acceptor type)

(iv) Chiral affinity with help of proteins (chymotrypsin and serum albumin)

(v)   Host-guest type of interactions within the chiral cavities (imprinted polymers and cyclodextrins).

The resolution of enantiomeric separation process is dependent upon the difference in steric fit, that is linked by hydrogen bonding of the solute molecules in the chiral environment. Some types of stationary phases are detailed below:

A. Derivatives of Polysaccharides

The D-glucose units of polysaccharides are linked by 1-4 glucosidic bonds, and they form a natural polymer with a helical structure. Strands around the chiral glucose can be formed by derivatising the three hydroxyls on each glucose unit. The derivatized glucose unit acts as a site with chiral nature and it discriminates between enantiomers that interrelate in a different way with the strands. The mobile phases for this type of stationary phases are organic solvents and aqueous solvents. Recently, phenyl carbamate derivatives of glucose and acetate ester are used as stationary phases of this class.

B. *Immobilized Proteins Containing Stationary Phases*

This type of stationary phases is one of the most widely used stationary phases in chiral chromatography and it involves the use of protein immobilized to the surface of support like silica gel. Several biomolecules with chiral nature have exhibited stereo selective affinity to proteins like a1-acid glycoprotein, and serum albumin. The mobile phases used for such stationary phases are aqueous buffers with minor amounts of organic modifiers. With efficient protein stationary phases slight variations in the affinities of the enantiomers to the protein affect the resolution between them. Ovomucoid and a-chymotrypsin are also immobilized on silica gel and can be used for analysis of various pharmaceutical compounds.

C. *Chiral Cavities*

One more method of separation on a stationary phase based on chirality is designing of chiral cavities, where there is stereoselective guest-host interaction that rules the resolution. The primary factor to be considered for retention and chiral recognition in this type of stationary phases is the exact fit of the molecule to the cavity with respect to the shape and size. Crown ethers, and cyclodextrins are examples of such type of stationary phases. The monomers are set such that a hollow condensed shaped cone is formed. A hydrophobic chiral cavity is developed with methylene and 1, 4 glucoside bonding, where the solute can interact. The exterior surface is hydrophilic in nature and is surrounded by hydroxyl groups. Mobile phases employed for such type of stationary phases are aqueous solutions mixed with organic solvents. In case of cyclodextrin stationary phases the mobile phases are aqueous and retention occurs due to inclusion complexation, where the a polar molecular segment is attracted to the a polar cavity. When aromatic groups are present, the interactions with the glucoside oxygens lead to stereo selective orientation in the cavity. When linear or acyclic hydrocarbons are concerned the positions in the cavity are occupied in a random fashion. It is necessary that the solute possesses at least a single aromatic ring, reversed phase mode is tried in chiral separation.

D. *Pirkle Type: p-donor p-acceptor Stationary Phases*

This type of chiral stationary phase was one of the oldest one used for analysis. The ground-breaking work of Pirkle made such a great contribution that the entire class of donor-acceptor type of stationary phases was named after him. The strands have a hydrogen bonding agent and dipole stacking inducing structure with a p-donor or p-acceptor aromatic fragment. The ground work started with the use of p-donor type anthryl groups, which were after wards changed to p-acceptor dinitro benzoylphenyl (DNBP) derivatives of amino acids. The success of DNBP initiated the growth of the field of chiral liquid chromatographic separations by means of chiral stationary phases. As the DNBP group is a p-acceptor, the solutes must have a p-donor group like an aromatic ring with ether, alkyl or amino substituents, so that the separation occurs. The solutes should have the ability to form hydrogen bonds with the amide group that is attached to an aromatic group on the stationary phase.

Applications of Chiral Chromatography

- To study chirality in pharmaceuticals: Biological interactions of chiral compounds including proteins, carbohydrates and enzymes have been studies with the help of chiral chromatography. Pharmacokinetic studies of enantiomers of drugs such as Ketoprofen, Propranolol, Ibuprofen and Warfarin.

- Assessment of risks and development of enantiomeric drugs: Chiral chromatography is used in identification of enantiomers that are excreted after metabolism of drugs in order to establish the safety, toxicity, pharmacokinetic and pharmacodynamic profile of the drugs.

- In eco-toxicological applications: Chiral chromatography is applied in the analysis of sludge for identification of antifungal compounds like econazole, miconazole and propiconazole, in analysis of compounds such as Fluoxetine in waste water effluent and influent, analysis of compounds such as Venlafaxine in laboratory scale bioreactors

- Chiral chromatography is applied in studies involving environmental biotransformation, analysis of water contamination with sewage, and sewage epidemiology.

10 Analysis of Data obtained from Hyphenated Chromatographic Techniques

Introduction

Traditional chromatographic separation criteria's or response functions are based upon chromatograms recorded by single-channel detectors. In the data of a chromatographic analysis when the peaks overlap there is a lack of information about all the chemical components and the peak purity. Such a data is a store of very important features of separation process and if not carefully interpreted it will lead to an erroneous and ambiguous evaluation of separation value. Nevertheless, if hyphenated chromatography spectroscopy instruments are assisted with chemometric methods the data that will be generated will increase the information content of the detection to a large extent. Such information, if appropriately utilised, can focus a new light on the quality of chromatographic separation.

Estimating the Number of Chemical Components

Estimating the number of chemical components with known experimental noise

Chen et al. suggested a method for estimation of the number of chemical components by analysis of the ratios of eigen values with the help of smoothed and ordinary (unsmoothed) PCA (RESO) of spectral data. Smoothed PCA (SPCA) enforces a roughness penalty on ordinary Principal Component Analysis. For Principal Components are interrelated to the real chemical components and the eigen vectors of a linear combination of smooth spectra are also smooth. Thus, these will be very slightly affected by the roughness penalty. The eigen values of a smoothed principal component analysis and Principal component analysis for chemistry-related Principal Components are very comparable; where as for Principal Components that are considered for the noise, the eigen vectors of a linear combination of noise factors are very rough. These principal components are thus very significantly affected by the roughness penalty, and so the eigen values of SPCA for noise factors are much lesser than those which are obtained by ordinary Principal component analysis. On the basis of this, RESO was defined as:

$$RESO = \frac{\lambda_i\left(SPCA\right)}{\lambda_i\left(PCA\right)}$$

There are many methods developed for the statistical estimation of the number of chemical components. Two empirical methods were proposed by Malinowski, the imbedded error (IE) and the factor indicator (IND) functions, which are defined as:

$$IE = \left(\frac{N\sum_j^p = N+1\lambda_j}{mp\left(p-N\right)}\right)^{1/2}$$

$$IND = \frac{RE}{\left(p-N\right)^2}$$

where, RE is the real error and RE = RSD

and RSD is given as:

$$RSD = \frac{1}{m\left(p-N\right)}\sum_{i=1}^{m}\sum_{j=1}^{p}\left(\overline{x}_{ij}^2 - x_{ij}^2\right) = \frac{1}{m\left(p-N\right)}\sum_{k=N+1}^{p}\lambda_k$$

where x_{ij} is the element in the 'i'th row and 'j'th column of the raw data matrix and $\overline{x}_{ij}$ is the corresponding element of the data matrix that is reconstructed with the first 'N' Principal Components.

It has been proved that if the errors are distributed evenly, IE will decrease with increased number of Principal Components and when the number of Principal components 'PCs' (N) exceeds the number of real chemical components (n), IE will begin to increase. Thus, one can determine the number of chemical components as the N yielding the minimum IE value. IND is a more insightful criterion than IE, as it can reach a clearer minimum, which can frequently appear even when IE has no minimum at all. Few studies have demonstrated satisfying performances of IND, but further analyses are stilled needed to completely understand this method and explain its significances.

Cross validation (CV) is also a method that can be used to determine the number of chemical components. For Cross validation, the reduced matrix is subjected to PCA by deleting the raw data matrix and finally the deleted part is tested using various numbers (N) of PCs and the prediction sum of squares (PRESS) of the errors is calculated with the equation mentioned below:

$$\mathrm{Press}(N) = \sum_{i=1}^{m} \sum_{j=1}^{p} \left(x_{ij} - \hat{x}_{ij}(N) \right)^2$$

where x_{ij} is the element in the 'i'[th] row and 'j'[th] column of the data matrix X and $\hat{x}_{ij}(N)$ is its predicted value by target test using N PCs. Certain criteria are necessary to determine the number of chemical components, when PRESS values are to be calculated for different numbers of PCs. Wold *et al.,* recommended that the number of chemical components must be the N that yields the global minimum PRESS value or the first local minimum.

Chemometric Methods for Estimation of Elution Sequence

There are two features which should be brought into consideration before introducing chemometric methods for the estimation of elution sequence of different components. The first feature is that, like many kinetic reaction systems, in a chromatographic separation the elution profiles vary with the retention times. Another important aspect of chromate-graphic process is that, similar to the potential of chromatography to separate various constituents, even the elution of different components exhibit common patterns of having distinct regions of chemical components, zero-component regions, and regions with varying number of chemical components. The elution patterns are often critical to obtain exclusive resolution of pure elution profiles and spectra and these can be easily obtained from rank graphs.

Maeder and co-workers proposed evolving factor analysis (EFA), based on the two features of chromatographic process mentioned above. In order to understand the application of this method, for a simulated 4-component system, we consider a two-way data set with spectral absorptions measured at 120 wavelengths recorded for 100 retention points by a hyphenated chromatography–spectroscopy instrument (Fig. 10.1(a)). The figure depicts the pure elution profiles and pure spectra of 4 chemical components. It should be assumed that the data set shown in Fig. 10.1a is a single data set available for analysis and (Fig. 10.2(b) depicts pure elution profiles and pure spectra, where as (Fig. 10.1(c)) can only be obtained by comprehensive self-modelling curveresolution (SMCR) or other methods, and they are represented here only to make comparison with the rank graph.

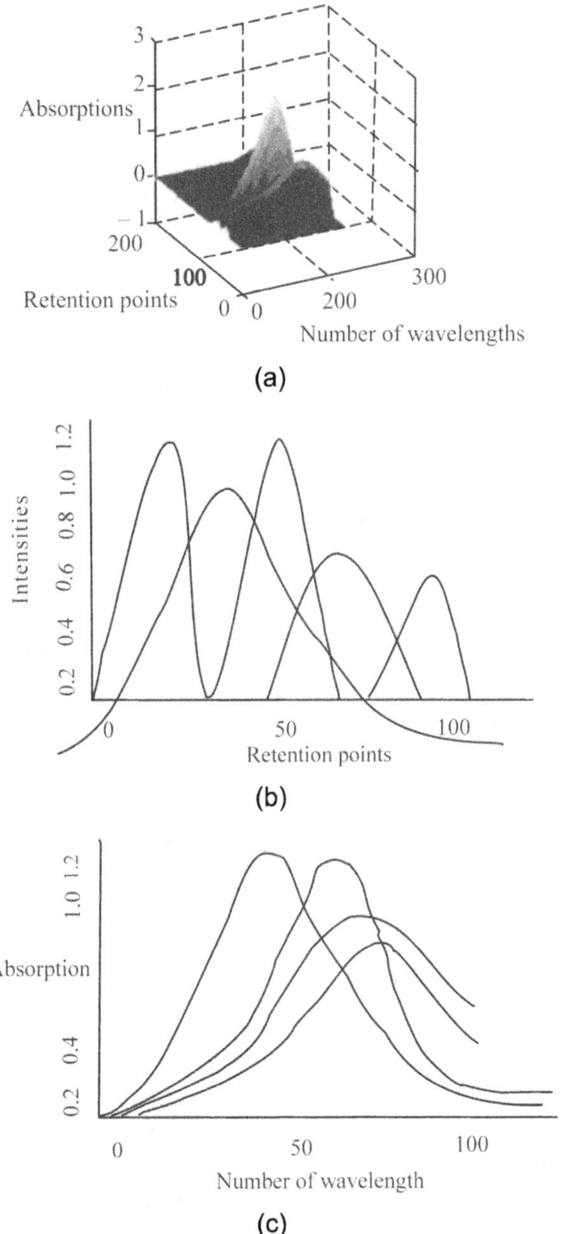

Figure 10.1 A. A simulated two-way data measurement, **B.** Elution profiles for four components, **C.** Pure spectra of components

EFA contains evolving Principal component analysis (PCA) along the retention points, in forward and backward direction. In the forward movement, one can perform PCA of m sub-matrices containing the spectra composed at retention points 1, 1 to 2, 1 to 3, 1 to 4 ..., 1 to m^{-1} and 1to m, where m is the total number of retention points. The logarithms of *eigen values* obtained from each PCA are plotted against the numbers of added retention points, namely, 1, 2, 3, 4, . . ., m^{-1} and m. (Characteristic values are also known as eigen values). As only the first N eigen values of the m times of a Principal Component Analysis are used and can be such ordered in an $N \times m$ matrix as below:

$$\begin{bmatrix} \lambda_{11},\lambda_{21},\lambda_{31},\lambda_{41},...,\lambda_{m1} \\ \lambda_{12},\lambda_{22},\lambda_{32},\lambda_{42},...,\lambda_{m2} \\ \lambda_{13},\lambda_{23},\lambda_{33},\lambda_{42}...,\lambda_{m3} \\ \vdots \\ \lambda_{1N},\lambda_{2N},\lambda_{3N},\lambda_{4N}...,\lambda_{mN} \end{bmatrix}$$

For this consideration, the number N should be greater than the total number of constituents. For N-1 matrices the total number of eigenvalues is less than N and zeros can be used to create N eigenvalues. In backward movement similarly, one can carry out the Principal Component Analysis of m sub-matrices containing the spectra collected at retention points m, m to m^{-1}, . . ., m to 2, and m to 1.

Merging the data of forward and backward PCA, we can determine the elution sequence of each chemical component. EFA is an effective method to sophisticatedly get the elution sequence by utilizing the evolutionary feature of chromatographic separation and it is used as a standard step for many SMCR methods till date.

Peak Purity Assessment

The objectives of analysts are the qualitative and quantitative analysis of components of interest. For qualitative analysis of unknown samples, the retention regions and the chemical components in the adjacent peaks that are present in the corresponding chromatographic peaks are considered. The evaluation of peak purity of the peaks is an indispensable step. The peak purity assessment includes the determination of impurities or minor components if present along with the major components.

Frenich et al. documented the use of three methods: simple to use interactive self-modelling mixture analysis (SIMPLISMA), orthogonal projection (OPA) and Needle Search (NS) for the estimation of the number of chemical compounds present in a complex multi-component system. In one of the SMCR methods, the simple-to-use interactive self-modelling mixture analysis (SIMPLISMA), at the 'i'th retention point, and the purity of the selected spectrum is defined as:

$$p_i = w_i \, \frac{\sigma_i}{\mu_i + \text{offset}}$$

Where σ_i and μ_i are the standard deviation and mean of each spectrum i, respectively. The offset is a percentage that is set to be 1-3% of the maximum mean value. This prevents the spectra with low mean intensities from obtaining high purity values. First, the weight w_i is set to be the square of the length of the normalized spectrum i. The spectra with the largest estimated purity values are selected as the "Purest spectra". With the help of SIMPLISMA one can update the selection of reference spectra, and the values of off sets. One can also estimate the weights and purity of the estimated peaks until the fitting error is approximately equal to the experimental noise. The number of selected spectra determines the number of chemical components.

OPA selects the first reference (pure) spectrum which has the highest estimated dissimilarity with the mean spectrum. The relationship of the dissimilarity of 'i'th spectrum with the mean spectrum is defined as:

$$D_i = \det\left(Y_i^T Y_i\right)$$

Where, "det" is the determinant of a matrix and columns of Yi consist of the 'i'th spectrum and normalized mean spectrum. As in SIMPLISMA, the reference spectra can then be selected one by one as the spectrum with the highest dissimilarity in addition to the previously selected reference spectra. The main advantage of OPA over SIMPLISMA is that OPA can detect an impurity from the first spectrum that is selected and that no normalization parameters are required.

Bibliography

1. De Juan, A., & Tauler, R. (2007). Factor analysis of hyphenated chromatographic data: exploration, resolution and quantification of multi component systems. Journal of Chromatography A, 1158(1), 184-195.

2. Archer J. P. Martin (1952). "The development of partition chromatography". Nobel Lecture, December 12, 1952. Nobel Lectures, Chemistry 1942-1962, Elsevier Publishing Company, Amsterdam, 1964.

3. Bauer G.K., and Kovar K.A., (1999) Direct HPTLC-FTIR online coupling: interaction of acids and bases with the binder in coated HPTLC plates. J. of Planar Chromatogr – Modern TLC, 11, 30-33.

4. Bernet, P., Blaser, D., Berger, S., & Schär, M. (2004). Development of a robust capillary electrophoresis–mass spectrometer interface with a floating sheath liquid feed. CHIMIA International Journal for Chemistry, 58(4), 196-199.

5. Bourne, S., Haefner, A. M., Norton, K. L., & Griffiths, P. R. (1990). Performance characteristics of a real-time direct deposition gas chromatography/Fourier transform infrared spectrometry system. *Analytical chemistry*, *62*(22), 2448-2452

6. Branley R.K, Bullock.D.G., (2004) Clarke's Analysis of Drugs and Poisons, 3rd Ed., Pharmaceutical Press, London Vol.1,161-171.

7. Burlingame.A.L., Boyd.R.K., Anal.Chem., 70 (1998) 647R.

8. Cazes.J., Raymond P. W., (2002), Chromatography Theory, Marcel Decker, Inc, NY, 443-454.

9. Van Noostr and Rheinhold, (1975). Chromatography: a laboratory handbook of chromatographic and electrophoretic techniques. Heftman, E. (Ed.), Co., New York.

10. Connors, K. A. (2007). A textbook of pharmaceutical analysis. John Wiley & Sons, 3rd Ed., Willey Interscience, New York, 373-438.

11. Das, Y. Sharif, A. Khan, P. Das, and S.M. Shaheen, (2002), Environ. Pollut., 120, 255

12. Dynamics of chromatography, (1965), Part 1, Principles and theory. Giddings, J.C., Keller, R.A. (Eds.), Marcel Dekker Inc., New York.

13. Ettre, L. S. (2001). "The Predawn of Paper Chromatography". Chromatographia, vol. 54, pp. 409-414.

14. Fried, J. Sherma, (1999), Thin-Layer Chromatography, Fourth Edition, Revised and expanded, Marcel Dekker Inc., New York - Basel, pp-499. ISBN 0-8247-0222-0.

15. G. Gubitz, (1990), "Separation of Drug Enantiomers by HPLC Using Chiral Stationary Phases- A Selective Review", Chromatographia, 30, 555-564.

16. G.A. Antonious, G.A. Patel, J.C. Snyder, and M.S. Coyne, (2004), J. Environ. Sci. Health B, 39, 19.

17. Giddings. J. C, (1965), Dynamics of Chromatography, Part I: Principles and Theory(Chromatographic Science Series Vol.1), Marcel Deckker, New York

18. Gratzfeld-Hüsgen and R. Schuster, (1996) HPLC for Food Analysis: A Primer, Hewlett-Packard, Palo Alto, Calif, USA, p.85.

19. Heftmann, E. (Ed.). (2004). Chromatography: Fundamentals and applications of chromatography and related differential migration methods-P, Applications. Elsevier, Volume 51, pp A1 -A68.

20. Heftman.E.,Chromatography, (2004), Fundamentals & applications of Chromatography and Related differential migration methods,6th Ed., Elsevier, Amsterdam, Vol. 69A, 253-291.

21. Hubschmann, H., (2001), Handbook of GC/MS: Fundamentals and Applications. Wiley-VCH Verlag, Germany.

22. ISO, pr EN ISO FDIS 15189,(2002). Medical Laboratories - Particular Requirements for Quality and Competence, Geneva, International Standards Organization,

23. J. Sherma, (2005), Pesticide Analysis by Thin Layer Chromatography. In: J. Cazes (ed.) Encyclopedia of Chromatography, 2nd edn, Marcel Dekker, New York, pp. 1230-1238

24. J.J. Kirkland and L.R. Snyder, (1974), American Chemical Society Short Course, "Solving Problems in Modern Liquid Chromatography.

25. Jinno, K., Nakanishi, S., & Nagoshi, T. (1984). Microcolumn gel permeation chromatography with inductively coupled plasma emission spectrometric detection. Analytical Chemistry, 56(11), 1977-1979.

26. Jinno K. (2001), Basics and applications of hyphenated-detection system in HPLC: Part I-Basics and applications in HPLC. Pharm Stage; 1:81-94.

27. José Manuel Amigo, Marta J. Popielarz, Raquel M. Callejón, Maria L. Morales, Ana M. Troncoso, Mikael A. Petersen, Torben B. Toldam-Andersen. (2010), Comprehensive analysis of chromatographic data by using PARAFAC2 and principal components analysis. Journal of Chromatography A, 1217, 4422-4429.

28. Krugers, J. (1968), Instrumentation in Gas Chromatography. Centrex Publishing Company-Eindhoven, Netherlands.

29. L.R. Snyder,(1978), "Classification of the Solvent Properties of Common Liquids", *J. Chromatogr. Sci.*, 16, 223-234.

30. Laurence M. Harwood, Christopher J. Moody. Experimental organic chemistry: Principles and Practice (Illustrated edition ed.). pp. 159–173. ISBN 978-0632020171.

31. Lesney, Mark S. (1998). "Creating a Central Science: A brief history of 'color writing'". Today's Chemist at Work, vol. 7, no. 8, pp. 71-72.

32. Lindon JC, Nicholson JK, Sidelmann UG, Wilson ID.(1997), Directly coupled HPLC-NMR and its application to drug metabolism. *Drug Metab Rev.*; 29:707-46.

33. M. Kastelan-Macan and S. Babic, Pesticides. In: J. Sherma and B. Fried, (2003), (eds) Handbook of Thin Layer Chromatography, 3rd edn, Marcel Dekker, New York, pp. 767–805.

34. Niessen WM. (1999), Liquid chromatography-Mass spectrometry. 2 nd ed. New York: Dekker; Albert K. On-line use of NMR detection in separation chemistry.

35. Nomenclature For Chromatography (IUPAC Recommendations 1993) Prepared for publication by L. S. ETI'REPure&Appl, Chem., Vol. 65, No. 4, pp. 81H72, (1993). Printed in Great Britain.©1993 IUPAC.

36. OECD, (1992), Good Laboratory Practice and Compliance Monitoring , Paris, OECD

37. Patel, R.B. and Patel, M.R. and Patel, B.G. (2011), Experimental Aspects and Implementation of HPTLC. In: Shrivastava, M.M. HPTLC. New York: Springer,; pp. 41- 54.

38. Pirkle W.H. and Pochapsky T.C., (1987), "Advances in Chromatography" eds. Giddings J.C., Grushka E. and Brown P.R., Marcel Dekker Inc. NY, vol 27, 73-127.

39. Remington's Pharmaceutical Sciences,(1990), 18th Ed., Mack Publishing Company, Pennsylvania , 1513 -1519.

40. Remington's Pharmaceutical Sciences, (1990), 18th edn., Mack Publishing Company, Pennsylvania , 529-554.

41. Rolf Manne, Bjørn-Vidar, (2000), Grande Resolution of two-way data from hyphenated chromatography by means of elementary matrix transformations. Chemometrics and Intelligent Laboratory Systems. 50, 35-46.

42. S. Jayaraman, M. Naika, and H. Das,(2003). J. Food Sci. Technol.-Mysore, 40, 319

43. S. Levin and S. Abu-Lafi, (1993), "The Role of Enantioselective Liquid Chromatographic Separations Using Chiral Stationary Phases in Pharmaceutical Analysis", in Advances in Chromatography. E. Grushka and P. R. Brown, Eds., Marcel Dekker Inc.: NY, Vol. 33,233-266.

44. Scott, R. P. W. (1996). Chromatographic Detectors: Design, Function, and Operation. Marcel Dekker, Inc., USA,

45. Scott. P. W, Liquid Chromatography Column Theory, John Willey and Sons, Chi Chester, 1-13.

46. Scott. P. W, (2001), Raymond, Encyclopedia of Chromatography, 10th Ed., Marcel Dekker, Inc. USA, 252-254.

47. Sherma. J., (2001), Encyclopedia of Pharmaceutical Technology, 2nd Ed., Marcel Dekker, Inc. USA, 252-254.

48. Shrivastava, M.M. (2011), An Overview of HPTLC: A Modern Analytical Technique with Excellent Potential for Automation, Optimization, Hyphenation, and Multidimensional Applications. In: Shrivastava, M.M. HPTLC. New York: Springer, pp. 3- 24.

49. Skoog A.D., West. D. M., Holler H.M.,(1996), Fundamentals of Analytical Chemistry,7th Ed., Saunders College Publishing, Vol.3, 1-10.

50. Skoog, D. A.; Holler, F. J.; Crouch, S. R. (2007), Principles of Instrumental Analysis. Sixth Edition, Thomson Brooks/Cole, USA.

51. Teresa Kowalska, Joseph Sherma, (2006),, Preparative Layer Chromatography, by   CRC Press, Taylor & Francis Group, Boca Raton, FL 33487-2742, ISBN 0-8493-4039-X.

52. Wilson ID, (2003), Brinkman UA. Hyphenation and hypernation: the practice and prospects of multiple hyphenation. *J. Chromatogr A.* 1000; 325s.